Monographs from the African Studies Centre,
Leiden

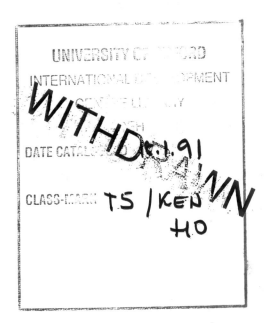

Intervention
in Child Nutrition

Intervention in Child Nutrition: Evaluation Studies in Kenya

Jan Hoorweg & Rudo Niemeijer

Kegan Paul International
London and New York

First published in 1989 by Kegan Paul International Limited
PO Box 256, London WC1B 3SW

Distributed by
International Thomson Publishing Services Ltd
North Way, Andover, Hants SP10 5BE
England

Routledge, Chapman and Hall Inc
29 West 35th Street
New York, NY 10001
USA

The Canterbury Press Pty Ltd
Unit 2, 71 Rushdale Street
Scoresby, Victoria 3179
Australia

Produced by Worts-Power Associates

Set in Times
by Wessex Typesetters
(Division of The Eastern Press Ltd)
Frome, Somerset
and printed in Great Britain
by Dotesios Printers Ltd
Trowbridge, Wiltshire

© Afrika-Studiecentrum 1989

ISBN 07103 0276-2

Contents

Acknowledgements

The studies that form the basis for this monograph were carried out between 1976 and 1979 and were made possible because of the support, co-operation and goodwill of many organizations. The African Studies Centre in Leiden has a standing interest in child nutrition and provided the funds and resources for what was ambitiously termed the 'Nutrition Intervention Research Project'. Three organizations in Kenya concerned with child nutrition generously allowed access to their clinics, as well as to their staff and programme participants: the Ministry of Health, the Ministry of Housing and Social Services and Catholic Relief Services. The project was associated with the University of Nairobi (Bureau of Educational Research) which formed our administrative base and provided us with office space and other amenities.

We wish to thank the responsible individuals at these organizations for their assistance which was instrumental in realizing the project: at the African Studies Centre, Prof. A. Kobben, the late Prof. J. Voorhoeve and, in particular, the General Secretary, G. Grootenhuis; at the Ministry of Health, Dr S. Kanani and Mrs S. Ngui; at the Ministry of Housing and Social Services, Dr G. Siboe, C. Ngari and Mrs M. Thuo; at Catholic Relief Services, Dr C. Capone, Dr R. Dugas and Mrs Karanja; and at the Bureau of Educational Research, Dr A. Maleche and Mrs A. Krystall. We also wish to mention the various field officers of these organizations who never tired of our presence and who assisted us wherever they could: the supervisors of Catholic Relief Services, the clinic personnel at the Pre-School Health clinics, the staff at the Family Life Training Centres as well as the individual Nutrition Field Workers. We must also mention the support received from the Medical Research Centre and its director, Dr Th. Haanegraaf; the Kigumo District Officer who made government living quarters available which served as our research house for the duration of the surveys; the staff of the Central Bureau of Statistics and the staff of the computer centre of the University of Nairobi who assisted with the first analysis of the data.

We are, of course, particularly obliged to our office staff and research assistants: Mr Wilson Kanyike, Mss Margaret Ng'ang'a, Rose Wanjira, Anne Gachui, Nelias Kanja, Josephine Kariuki, Josephine Muiruiri, Jane Waithira, Alice Wambui, Grace Wambui, Virginia Wambui, Nancy Wanjiru, and Irene Mburu. They provided invaluable help and shared many ups and downs with us and it is regrettable that projects such as this are only of limited duration. It was a good team.

Although the present monograph is authored by the two researchers with overall responsibility, several colleagues have participated in the project. Wil van Steenbergen assisted us with her experience of nutrition surveys; Henk Meilink collected the socio-economic data on the three districts; Elizabeth Githinji, our counterpart, greatly strengthened our field team; Ros Howie helped out with data collection at a difficult time; Marian Geuns assisted with the analysis of food consumption data. We also wish to thank the members of the advisory committee: Prof. J. Hautvast, the late Prof. J. Jaspars and Prof. J.P. Stanfield for their support and advice and we are grateful for the detailed comments on this manuscript by Prof. Jane Kusin and Ted Kliest.

In January 1981 the preliminary results of the studies were presented to the personnel of the organizations concerned at a two-day seminar. We are grateful for the favourable reception of the studies at the time and wish to acknowledge the various comments by the seminar participants.

The detailed analysis and reporting of data required further assistance, notably of the staff of the Computer Centre of Leiden University; of Ina Rike, our patient English editor; and of the office staff at the African Studies Centre: Bert Dubbeldam, Mieke Zwart, Adrienne v. Wijngaarden and Ria v. Hal. Nelly de Vink drew the maps.

Finally we wish to thank those individuals who did not find a place in the above summing-up but whose contributions we certainly appreciate: the late Dr D. Blankhart, Prof. J. Bennett, Prof. N. Bwibo, P. Dasen, J.G. and Mrs F. Grootenhuis, V. Hazard, H. Herr, H. Hesp, J. Hitchings, Dr A. Jansen, Prof. J. Kagia, L. v.d. Laan, S. Lakhani, J. Leeuwenburg, W. Klaver, E. Krystall, J. McDowell, Mrs Mimani, J. v. Luyk, J. Nijssen, J. Otieno, Ir. A. Parzer, K. Roesch, E. Ruchiami, R. Sarnoff, N. Scotney, Prof. M. Segall, Ch. Smith, L. Wasonga, Prof. M. Were and C. Worthman.

List of Boxes

List of Maps

List of Tables

List of Figures

Chapter 1

Introduction

The growing awareness of the nutritional problems in many developing countries, particularly on the African continent, has resulted in manifold nutrition interventions. Because of the substantial resources involved, either in the form of food aid, manpower, financial or other assistance, there is also a growing demand for evaluation of nutrition programmes on the part of both recipient and donor countries. For many years there was a tendency to relegate evaluation to a backseat position and evaluation of nutrition programmes was, in fact, something of a neglected art. Neglected because officers responsible for and charged with the daily management of nutrition programmes are mostly very practical people, aware of existing problems and equally aware of measures that need to be taken. Pressed by practical demands they often – understandably – feel that evaluation is too slow a process which, in the end, may not even produce conclusive results or concrete recommendations. The evaluation requirements, such as pre-testing of measuring instruments, pilot surveys, delineation of study conditions and selection of index and possible control children are elaborate and time-consuming. This is not to argue that evaluators are overly cautious in their approach. They, in their turn, are confronted with many different cultural settings and with programmes that often have unclear objectives, lack basic information, do not keep adequate records and are difficult to distinguish from other influences on child nutrition. Yet, they still have to come up with useful suggestions and are generally expected to make the best of a very difficult job. Over the past ten years, however, the need for evaluation has increasingly been recognized. Programme officials no longer ignore evaluation, rather they have the task of balancing the need for evaluation against the resources that can be set aside for evaluation purposes and the degree of interference with day-to-day activities that is acceptable. These are often difficult decisions and the quality of the evaluation is directly dependent on them.

Assessing the impact of nutrition intervention programmes is notoriously complicated because of the difficulty of distinguishing between the impact of the actual programmes and the influence of other factors. This is further complicated because many evaluations do not or cannot take the cultural characteristics of different groups of recipients into account. Consequently, impact studies are often inconclusive because of methodological weaknesses or because of lack of sensitivity, in which case possible effects may escape notice. In their efforts to gain control over external factors, many researchers call for more and more elaborate research designs, thus making the effort increasingly expensive. Such elaborate designs sometimes make matters even worse, because the demands of the design may alter the nature of the programme and, thereby, invalidate the evaluation at the same time. Other researchers, in response to the same problem, draw the opposite conclusion and advocate a relaxation of statistical rigour and more modest evaluation objectives. In fact, the topic has become something of an independent area of research by itself; witness several recent bibliographies and handbooks (Burgess, 1982; Figa-Talamanca, 1985; Klein et al., 1979; Sahn et al., 1984; Schurch, 1983).

In general there is a dilemma between sophisticated experimental research and post-facto evaluations that are more restricted in nature. In the first case, every effort is made to eliminate all possible distorting factors, and this usually requires that the evaluation be designed and included from the very beginning of the programme, often at great cost and effort. Such evaluation is usually justified as a one-time activity that can provide essential knowledge on the actual, but more often the potential achievements of a particular intervention. Alternatively there are post-facto evaluations, with a more down-to-earth approach, of programmes that have already been in operation for years. This kind of evaluation does not strive after experimental perfection, but aims to provide insights into certain programme effects, or into selected aspects of a programme. Usually this type of evaluation is less obtrusive in nature, and may therefore better reflect the achievements of a programme under actual field conditions.

The studies in this monograph follow this latter approach. Together they demonstrate a methodology of programme evaluation which is relatively simple and adapted to the conditions presented by many nutrition programmes in developing countries. Although the emphasis is on the use of comparatively simple designs, a satisfactory degree of sensitivity was realized through careful selection of index and control groups, and collecting data of a straightforward nature, with particular attention to accurate data collection.[1]

Initial studies that were carried out in Uganda were mainly of the nature of methodological trials, although there too attention focused on programmes under different conditions, notably the difference between a rural and urban environment. The results of these studies have been published in an earlier monograph (Hoorweg & McDowell, 1979).

Further studies were undertaken in Kenya between 1976 and 1979, under the title of Nutrition Intervention Research Project (NIRP). Like many African countries, Kenya covers a wide variety of ecological conditions, ranging from desert to fertile highlands, with all kinds of variations in between. Kenya's population at the time of the latest census in 1979 was 15.3 million, and it was expected to pass 20 million by 1985 (CBS, 1981b; 1983a). Three quarters of the landsurface of the country is considered unsuitable for agriculture with the consequence that the large majority of the population lives in that quarter of the country that is suitable for rainfed agriculture. There are three regions with major population concentrations: the central, western and coastal parts of the country. Kenya is one of the few countries which, in contrast to most African countries, cannot easily accommodate a much larger population (ICIHI, 1985). The country, however, has one of the highest rates of population growth in the world, estimated at 4% annually (World Bank, 1986), and pressure on land is becoming a problem in many places.

At the time when the present studies were initiated (early 1976),

3

there was little information on the nutritional status of children in Kenya. A number of incidental studies, though, were available and these had been brought together in a review by Blankhart (1974a).[2] Since then the Central Bureau of Statistics has held three national nutrition surveys among the rural population (CBS, 1977; 1979a; 1983b). The percentage of children with a low weight-for-age (below 80) was 33%, 25% and 23% in 1977, 1978 and 1983 respectively, although the figures are not strictly comparable because of differences in sample compositions.[3] The percentage of stunted children, with an H-A below 90, ranged from 24% to 29%; the percentage of severely wasted children (W-H below 80) varied between 3% and 5%. These rates of malnutrition and undernutrition are moderate compared with the figures reported for Asian and Sahel countries (Brink et al., 1978; Kardjati et al., 1977; IDRC, 1981), but they are comparable with the rates reported for other Sub-Saharan countries such as Cameroon, Liberia and Sierra Leone (USAID, 1976; 1978a; 1978b).

The national figures, though, hide important variations within the population. There are differences in the rate of undernutrition in the various provinces of the country and differences have also been reported to exist between populations living in different ecological zones. Moreover, there are important differences in nutrition and nutritional status between children from different income groups and certain underprivileged groups exhibit high incidences of malnutrition.

At the time there were – and there still are today – a large number of nutrition programmes in Kenya. Many of these programmes consisted of incidental activities of agencies and even individuals, as such severely restricted in scope and coverage, and often temporary. There were only three programmes, apart from the national School Feeding Programme, which had a nationwide coverage and centralized organization (PBFL/FAO, 1973): the Nutrition Field Worker Programme of the Ministry of Health, the Pre-School Health Programme of Catholic Relief Services, and the Family Life Training (FLT) centres of the Department of Social Services. The three programmes represent quite different kinds of interventions: nutrition education, food supplementation and nutrition rehabilitation respectively.

Nutrition Field Workers are nurses who function as members of the maternal and child health (MCH) teams at government health centres. Their principal tasks are to monitor children under

4

five years of age and identify malnourished children for special attention, with an emphasis on providing nutrition education to the mothers attending government MCH services. The Pre-School Health (PSH) Programme is a food supplementation programme aimed at young children of families in needy circumstances. Once children are enrolled in the programme, mothers are expected to pay monthly visits to the centres until the child reaches the age of five years. FLT centres closely resemble what are internationally known as nutrition rehabilitation centres. Women with malnourished children are admitted for a period of about three weeks and are taught how to prepare a balanced diet and treat the condition of their children.

Because of their national coverage these programmes have to operate under the extreme diversity of circumstances typical of many African countries. These include ecological variation, ranging from arid lands to fertile highlands, but also include cultural differences, from the eating habits of pastoral peoples with a milk diet to those of agriculturalists dependent on cereals, roots or tubers as staple foods. Often these ecological and cultural differences are compounded, although this is not always the case, and the implications of these differences for the functioning and the impact of programmes is usually a matter of guesswork.

In order to neutralize the possible influence of cultural differences on programme impact, the studies were conducted at various locations in Central Province. This province, together with parts of Eastern Province, forms the population cluster of central Kenya. The province is characterized by sizeable variations in altitude, temperature and rainfall, resulting in considerable ecological diversity. In all, 70% of the surface area is considered suitable for farming. The population of the province was 2.3 million in 1979 and consists mainly of one ethnic group, the Kikuyu. The majority of the inhabitants are concentrated on the mid-slopes of the mountain ranges: an area with a very high population density, at least by African standards. In this sense conditions in Central Province are almost certainly a precursor of conditions as they will sooner or later arise elsewhere in Kenya, in high potential areas with increasing population pressure.

The studies in this volume were aimed at evaluating the impact of different types of nutrition intervention among rural populations, together with the implications that variations in ecology and household circumstances have for the impact of the programmes. The three programmes described above were selected as the object of study because they were ongoing programmes that had proved to be viable, unlike so many pilot or experimental projects that perished as soon as they were left to their own devices. By the nature of our interest the studies concentrated on impact evaluation, and followed the unobtrusive, low-key procedures outlined above (NIRP, 1976; 1978). This means that the degree of control over various other factors influencing child nutrition was often limited, that ad hoc solutions had sometimes to be found for various methodological complications, and that conclusions could only be drawn with a certain amount of caution – caution too not to dismiss lightheartedly the efforts of programme staff who often perform their work under very difficult and frustrating circumstances. Consequently we felt justified in taking a positive view of any indications of success, however modest.

The findings of the studies were presented in a series of project reports with specific recommendations for each programme (Hoorweg & Niemeijer, 1980a, 1980b, 1982). These reports serve as the primary means to make the statistical data available and the reader should consult them if more detailed information is required. This book is not so much concerned with a detailed presentation of the data, but rather with comparing the different studies, bringing them together in one publication, putting them in a more general perspective and drawing general conclusions. It is, first and foremost, an account of impact evaluation of nutrition programmes: its ideal practice in contrast to its actual implementation, the inherent methodological complications and the practical limitations under field conditions.

Chapter 2

Nutrition Intervention & Evaluation

2.1 Intervention in Child Nutrition

Nutrition interventions are of many kinds, difficult to cast in a single conceptual framework. Some interventions are general in nature; agrarian reforms or improvements of marketing systems, for example, aim only indirectly at improving the nutrition of the population, and economic objectives usually have the first priority. Other interventions aim more directly at increasing food availability to the population. Food-price subsidies, for instance, aim to improve the food entitlement of certain sections of the population, and at the same time guarantee national food production by keeping producer prices attractive. Storage loss prevention concentrates on the preservation of foodstocks to increase food availability either at subsistence level or for marketing purposes. Food fortification is another type of intervention, aimed at improving the quality of the diet through addition of certain scarce nutrients to suitable foodstuffs. Finally, of course, there is the massive food aid that we have witnessed over the past decade. All these interventions have in common that they concentrate primarily on food provision and food availability, and aim either to increase food production, to provide food or nutrients by other means, or to achieve a better distribution of available foods among the population.

In contrast, interventions in child nutrition generally focus more on food consumption and are often aimed at individual cases, usually involving direct contact between programme staff and mothers and children. Even so, there exist considerable variations between different types of intervention in child nutrition – notably variations in type of approach, nature of the target group and programme objectives. Different authors have classified child nutrition programmes in slightly different ways. Beaton & Bengoa (1976) in their handbook on nutrition in preventive medicine devote separate chapters to nutritional surveillance, nutrition education, supplementary feeding and nutrition rehabilitation. Austin & Zeitlin (1981) in a later handbook on nutrition intervention in developing countries, reserve separate chapters for supplementary feeding, nutrition education and integrated nutrition and health care. Since nutritional surveillance and integrated nutrition and health care usually consist of a composite of measures, three basic forms of nutrition intervention can be distinguished: nutrition education, food supplementation and nutrition rehabilitation.

Nutrition education in developing countries is aimed at the improvement of food-related practices, but is usually concerned with the improvement of individual food consumption, more in particular that of small children (Bosley, 1976; Zeitlin & Formacion, 1981). Although the education effort can be directed at different audiences, such as policy makers, health professionals and teachers (groups that can in turn influence present and future generations of mothers), nutrition education is most commonly aimed at housewives or mothers, for self-evident reasons. The different forms of nutrition instruction range from mass media and formal education to posters and booklets, but it is usually agreed that instruction is most effective when given to individuals or to small groups. Education is often included as part of other interventions, thus securing access to an existing audience.

In rural areas in developing countries the teaching often focuses on the introduction of new practices and better utilization of existing household resources. To combat harmful nutritional practices may also be an objective of the intervention, although this is usually a less important aspect than is often thought. Zeitlin &

Formacion (1981: 59) give an interesting list of common harmful food and health beliefs in different countries, pointing out at the same time that most of these beliefs have potential beneficial functions as well. Preferably teaching is adapted to local practices and available food resources, characterized by active audience participation and proceeding in small steps, with the consequence that it will take considerable time for any effects of the instruction to become visible. Although a general increase in research attention for nutrition education has been noted in Western countries (Gussow & Contento, 1984), this is far less so in the case of Third World countries. Although nutrition education is often regarded as an important component of rural development, the resources and manpower actually allocated to it are usually modest, and knowledge about the conditions which make for success or failure of nutrition education in the rural areas of developing countries is still very limited (Sinclair & Howatt, 1980).

Supplementary feeding consists of the provision of foods, free of charge or at low cost, to vulnerable groups to cover deficiencies in their normal diet (Bailey & Raba, 1976; Scrimshaw, 1982). The main forms of food supplementation in developing countries are programmes for pre-school children, pregnant and lactating women, school children, and also industrial workers. A major part of the international funds for nutrition are, in fact, spent on supplementary feeding programmes, and it was estimated that in 1979 over 50 million children received some kind of food supplement (Anderson et al., 1981: 25). Supplementary feeding of children usually takes the form of on-site feeding or take-home programmes; nutrition rehabilitation centres are sometimes also included under this heading. In the early years after 1945, the main item of food supplementation was milk as an important source of protein. More recently, with the growing realization that caloric deficiency is frequently more severe than protein deficiency as such, programmes generally try to offer a balance between high protein and high calorie foods. There is also a growing trend to utilize more local foods instead of imported food commodities, if at all possible. Estimates of the costs of supplementation vary but for the take-home and on-site programmes the costs per child are generally estimated at between $10 and $30 per annum (Anderson et al., 1981).

The term nutrition rehabilitation is usually reserved for the treatment of severe cases of protein-energy malnutrition. Treatment can be given in the form of hospital admission or at nutrition rehabilitation centres (Bengoa, 1976). Experiences with hospital treatment often have not been positive, mortality rates are high, hospitalization is usually lengthy, and the number of relapses tends to be high (Cook, 1971; Bengoa, 1976). This has led to a search for alternatives, notably the treatment of malnourished children in nutrition rehabilitation centres: either day-care centres or residential centres. At day-care centres, children are brought daily for several hours, long enough to be given several meals. These centres represent a form of on-site feeding, the difference with supplementary feeding programmes being one of degree. Rehabilitation centres of the residential type require more staff and equipment and are more costly because children and mothers usually stay at the centres for a period of several weeks. A characteristic of nutrition rehabilitation is that mothers are closely involved in feeding their children back to health using locally available foods and indigenous cooking methods (Cutting, 1983). Nutrition rehabilitation centres have been introduced in many countries and have been evaluated on several occasions (Beaudry-Darisme & Latham, 1973; Beghin & Viteri, 1973). The costs of day-care centres have been estimated at about $0.50 per child per day or about $10.00 for three weeks (Bengoa, 1976). The costs of residential centres are higher: in Kenya, for example, they were estimated at $40.00 per child for a period of three weeks (HN, 1982), but this is still below the costs of hospital treatment. The limitations are that the coverage of nutrition rehabilitation centres is usually small compared with existing needs and that, especially day-care centres, are not particularly well suited for scattered rural populations.

Usually interventions in child nutrition consist of the following main elements: nutrition instruction, food supplementation and nutrition rehabilitation. Individual programmes differ considerably as to the form that these components or their possible combination may take. Programmes further differ regarding a number of secondary intervention characteristics, such as the nature of the target group, the type of contact with participants, the extent of monitoring of the nutritional status of children and the nature of any accompanying public health measures.

Nutrition intervention can be aimed at the general population, but the nature of most programmes is such that they are aimed at selected populations. Nutrition education is often aimed at mothers of young children, usually in combination with selected health measures such as immunization. For other interventions such as nutrition rehabilitation and supplementary feeding the key target groups are usually children between the ages of 6 and 48 months (and pregnant and lactating women). Within these groups certain cases sometimes receive priority; in the case of young children these are usually the children that show overt signs of protein-energy malnutrition, or that fall below certain weight criteria. Alternatively selection can also be done on the basis of social-economic indicators, notably household characteristics such as level of resources and family composition (Anderson et al., 1981). The actual targeting, however, is complicated and the danger exists of including cases that are not really in need of the intervention measures, or conversely, of excluding from the programme cases that require assistance. In practice programmes are faced by a trade-off between these two kinds of errors, the error of inclusion and the error of exclusion. Measures that lower the risk of the former, notably the tightening of admission procedures, usually lead to an increase in the latter type of error and vice versa. Much depends, however, on the prevalence of malnutrition in the population. Where prevalence is high it appears that efforts to discriminate among children and/or families are less effective than among populations where prevalence is low (Timmons et al., 1983; 1986).

Programmes vary considerably with regard to the frequency, intensity and duration of contact, i.e. the exposure of participants. Duration of contact can range from a relatively short period of some weeks, to a period of a few months, to extended periods of several years. Contacts of short duration are sometimes of greater intensity or frequency, such as in-patient care where children are under supervision for 24 hours a day, but not always as, for example, where an intervention merely accompanies an immunization campaign, in which case most children are seen on a few occasions only. The frequency of contact may also differ: it can be regular as in the case of on-site feeding and take-away programmes, or irregular as in the case of intervention through health centres where contact occurs mainly during consultations for illness. In general, programmes designed for high frequency of contact are of limited duration, whereas when duration is prolonged the frequency of contact tends to be less. There is often considerable difference between planned exposure and the exposure actually realized. In practice, mothers and children often drop out at an early stage, while the visits during the actual period of contact may be less frequent than planned.

Because child growth usually slows down long before a child becomes malnourished and since the reverse – regular weight gain – signifies healthy development, growth monitoring is an important diagnostic tool. Growth monitoring usually consists of regular weighing and recording of weights on a child growth chart in conjunction with nutrition advice, and the use of these charts is becoming increasingly widespread. More than 200 different growth charts are estimated to be currently in use, in over 80 countries (UNICEF, 1985). Growth monitoring has three functions: firstly to diagnose early those children requiring attention, secondly to supervise cases already participating in nutrition programmes, and thirdly to create awareness of child growth on the part of the parents. The effectiveness of monitoring depends, of course, on the frequency of contact, whether it is an occasional examination during a visit to a health centre, or the monthly weighing which is more or less the norm in many nutrition programmes. In fact, sometimes the weighing is regarded as the primary intervention, and other components, notably nutrition education, as secondary (Siswanto, Kusnanto & Rohde, 1980).

In support of the nutrition intervention as such most programmes also pay attention to public health aspects such as preventive health care, hygiene and family planning (Cook, 1976; Austin et al., 1981). The well known synergism between malnutrition and childhood infections, necessitates preventive measures: immunization and hygiene, especially sanitation and proper handling of drinking water and food. The form these measures take may differ: sometimes the programme personnel themselves provide immunization, in other cases participants may be referred to other departments or other health agencies. In that case, the actual effort amounts to little more than health instruction. In fact, the attention paid to hygienic measures usually consists of little more than advice, except in the case of an integrated nutrition and primary health care programme, that actively seeks to improve sanitation and water supply. The inclusion of family planning in nutrition programmes is more controversial; in some countries attention to family planning may make a programme unacceptable to large sections of the population.

Finally, mention should be made of nutrition surveillance. In its general sense nutritional surveillance systems involve data collection for national planning purposes, with data being drawn mostly from already existing sources. The systems include widely differing areas of information such as weather conditions, agricultural production projections, food prices and the nutritional status of the population. Routine monitoring of the nutritional state of young children is a part of nutritional surveillance, and is sometimes referred to as nutritional screening (Habicht & Mason, 1983; Mason et al., 1984). A few countries have a nationwide system whereby children are seen at health centres where their nutritional status is monitored. Children who appear to be failing are referred to (weekly or monthly) nutrition clinics at the same health centres, where mothers are given nutrition instruction and can be issued food rations. In case children still do not improve, they can ultimately be referred to nutrition rehabilitation centres.

2.2 Evaluation: Concepts & Definitions

Given the range of possible interventions and the different combinations of possible elements it is not surprising that the actual implementation and effectiveness of nutrition programmes show equally large variations. This is where the need for evaluation arises. In its broadest sense, evaluation concerns any information about operations and impact of programmes or policies. In this sense it may consist of the fleeting impressions of visiting experts as well as of hard empirical evidence (Hennigan et al., 1979). Evaluation has different functions. Firstly it serves as feedback to programme personnel about their performance and achievements; secondly, it provides information for national governments and international agencies about the way resources are utilized. It further serves to improve programme performance, and also to gain insights that can be used in the planning of future programmes. The extent to which each or all of these aims are indeed realized depends on the scope and thoroughness of the evaluation and, of course, depends on the different needs that agencies may have and the specific questions they want the evaluation to answer. Generally programme outcomes can only be expected in the long run and are difficult to measure because of the intervening time period, but many evaluations have tended to be scanty in coverage, biased, and conducted on an ad hoc basis (Allen & Koral, 1982).

This book is concerned with evaluation in a research sense, as a systematic effort to collect empirical evidence that is (at least in principle) open to verification and replication. An important distinction that needs to be mentioned here is that between process and impact evaluation, similar to the less used distinction between formative and summative evaluation. This terminology refers to the conceptual difference between the services offered by the programme and the actual effects or impact of the programme. Process (formative) evaluation is concerned with implementation, i.e. the degree and manner in which the planned services are indeed delivered. Impact (summative) evaluation is concerned with effects, i.e. the changes that the programme actually achieves. The first kind of evaluation is the more simple and easy to realize, the second is the more complex and relies heavily on research methods drawn from the social sciences (Box A).

In the case of fortification programmes (addition of nutrients to certain foods), process evaluation will concentrate on the production and distribution of the fortified foods and the extent of fortification that is realized. In the case of formulated foods or processed weaning foods for children from low-income populations, the actual production and distribution of the foods is the subject of process evaluation. In the case of education programmes, process evaluation assesses the frequency of educational activities, the number of personnel employed, the number of people reached, and so on. Process evaluation can also include cost assessment, either of overall costs or more specific calculation of the costs to supply a certain unit of service. This is sometimes referred to as cost-effectiveness calculation, although this is not strictly correct, because cost-effectiveness should include some measure of impact.

Impact evaluation in the case of food fortification and formulated foods seeks to establish whether the nutritional condition of individual recipients indeed improves, and also the extent to which such improvements actually occur among the population at large. For example, in the case of deficiency syndromes, such as goitre, to what extent the prevalence of the condition among the population decreases. Impact evaluation of supplementary feeding ascertains how the foods are utilized in practice; impact evaluation of nutrition education whether mothers adapt their nutritional practices, and

14

Box A. **Terminological confusion**

Because evaluation is a relatively recent area of interest, there are considerable differences in the use of terminology. This confusion is even more pronounced than usual with a new area of research because of the direct interest that many agencies have in the evaluation of their activities. The generally loose use of the term evaluation and the fact that some terms have changed meaning over the past years easily lead to confusion. The terms process evaluation and monitoring are cases in point.

Suchman (1967) distinguished between assessment of effort, assessment of performance and assessment of process, in that order. The term process indicated an analysis in depth of the intervention, i.e. how and why observed effects were achieved. This is now generally called impact evaluation, while the term process evaluation now mainly refers to the delivery of services, i.e. what Suchman termed assessment of effort. The present usage of the terms process and impact evaluation has a drawback in that it obscures the distinction between narrowly defined research on impact and research intended to provide more knowledge on the reasons behind the relative success or failure of an intervention. Instead, some authors now refer to 'special studies' (Sahn, 1985).

The term monitoring is mainly used to refer to the routine recording of, for example, staff activities, programme output or the condition of participants. The term however takes a rather twisted meaning in 'performance monitoring', where reference is made to routine data collection for purposes of impact evaluation (Gotzmann, 1986). Similarly it is doubtful whether a distinction between effect and impact, with the suggestion that the first is easier to measure than the second, helps to clarify thinking.

---

in both cases whether there is indeed an improvement in the nutritional status of the children concerned. The scope of impact evaluation may differ substantially. It may be limited to assessment of the desired, final outcomes of the intervention, usually the improved nutritional status of children. In that case the evaluation will often give little more than a strict indication of the degree of success. Impact evaluation may, however, also pay substantial attention to what are often called intermediate outcomes, such as changes in nutritional cognition of mothers or food consumption of children, in which case more insight can be gained into the possible reasons for success or failure.[1]

2.3 Impact Evaluation of Child Nutrition Programmes

Definitions of impact evaluation generally include reference to the measurement of programme effects by objective and systematic means. The term 'objective' refers to the use of reliable measuring instruments with standard routines; the term 'systematic' to the comparison of different groups of recipients (and non-recipients) in such a way that it reveals the impact of intervention, irrespective of other factors that influence child nutrition. Impact evaluation therefore has two major components: the indicators selected to reflect programme impact, and the design used for the comparison of different groups of recipients.

Indicators can, in principle, consist of very different measuring instruments, provided they reflect a meaningful aspect that the intervention aims to influence. In the case of child nutrition programmes they usually consist of some aspect of nutritional cognition and nutrition behaviour of mothers, or food consumption and nutritional status of children. Generally they may include the following:

(a) nutritional cognition (nutritional knowledge, nutritional attitudes);
(b) nutritional practices (food production, food storage, food preparation, food distribution);
(c) food consumption (dietary practices, food intake);
(d) nutritional status (anthropometry, clinical examination, biochemical indicators).

Since improvements in nutritional status are usually the desired outcome of intervention and are often regarded as the 'final' outcome, many impact evaluations have been limited to assessment of anthropometry. As mentioned above, this offers a very restricted form of impact evaluation. In the cases where programmes are not successful and no improvements in nutritional status are observed, it is often not possible to discover the exact reason for this failure, i.e. whether it is due to inadequate intervention methods, poor programme implementation or perhaps to hindering social influences. Moreover, in all programmes, however successful, there is usually a minority of cases that do not make good progress. Often there is an urgent need to know why these children do not improve, and it is difficult to discover the reason if data collection has been limited to nutritional status. It is therefore often advisable to include measures of other, intermediate, outcomes as well. A distinction is generally drawn between proximal and distal outcomes. In the case of nutrition education, a proximal outcome would be improved nutritional cognition and nutrition behaviour of the mothers. Improvements in nutritional status are more distal and the more distal the outcome the larger the potential array of variables that also influence it. By covering different indicators it is possible to test and compare alternative causal explanations or different causal pathways (Beaton, 1982).

It is usual to distinguish between treatment variables (various forms of nutrition intervention), non-treatment variables (other determinants of nutrition behaviour and nutrition status), and outcome variables (the proximal and distal outcomes). The major function of research designs is the control of non-treatment variables (also called confounding variables, nuisance variables, background variables or extraneous variables). Control to ensure that other determinants of nutrition behaviour and nutritional status do not offer rival explanations for any purported relation between treatment and outcome – control, furthermore to reduce residual variance to increase the power or sensitivity of the evaluation. Three different approaches to the control of variables exist: experimental control, quasi-experimental designs and statistical control (Hennigan et al., 1979).

Experimental control is realized by means of experimental designs: measures of outcome variables are compared across two or more groups of people who have received different amounts of treatment. These groups are formed by randomization, that is, random assignment of persons so that groups are equivalent in every respect except treatment. Any differences in outcomes can therefore be imputed to the effect of the treatment.

Quasi-experimental designs also involve comparisons between different treatment groups and control groups not exposed to treatment. Unlike in experimental designs, these groups are not

17

formed by random assignment and are 'non-equivalent' (Campbell & Stanley, 1966; Cook & Campbell, 1979). This leaves room for alternative explanations of any relations between treatment and outcome but this can be countered in a number of ways; notably by including non-treatment variables in the design, by excluding cases responsible for non-equivalence or by statistical adjustments. Each of these procedures, however, has drawbacks of its own; complicated designs, loss of generality of findings or large samples and long questionnaires being required.

While experimental and quasi-experimental designs make use of comparison groups, statistical control is characterized by statistical adjustment to remove the influence of non-treatment variables on outcome variables (Kerlinger, 1973; Cooper & Weekes, 1983). Statistical control uses the actual, observed correlations between variables and thus has the advantage of being more flexible because many research decisions can be left till the stage of data analysis, when the actual, observed relations between relevant variables can be taken into account.

In general, control over non-treatment variables is best achieved through randomization (i.e. experimental control). Both statistical control and quasi-experimental designs are flawed in the sense that there always remains the possibility that variables not included in the design or analysis contribute to results observed. Statistical control is generally considered superior to quasi-experimental designs because it gives more opportunity to remove residual variance. A further complication with impact evaluation of child nutrition programmes is the fact that the unit of study may differ within the context of one programme. For example, behaviour improvements will be expected of the mother, but improvements in nutritional status have to be measured among the children. In such cases it is often necessary to use different designs for different levels of analysis, i.e. among the children, the mothers or the households.

Most evaluations rely on quasi-experimental designs. A recent bibliography on nutrition education in Third World communities (Schurch & Wilquin, 1982), for example, shows that very few evaluations of nutrition education programmes relied on randomization or statistical control (Hoorweg, 1983). The reasons for this are fairly obvious. In the case of ongoing programmes it is difficult to allocate subjects randomly to different groups for ethical as well as practical reasons. A further complication with experimental designs is that it is necessary to study and compare the groups before as well as after treatment. Since nutrition programmes generally do not show any rapid effects such studies must necessarily cover extended periods of time. Not only do long-time periods in themselves present a practical research problem, they also make it more difficult to keep the different groups separate. Statistical control, on the other hand, requires advance knowledge about the determinants of nutrition behaviour and nutritional status but such knowledge for Third World communities is limited. Other complicating factors are that statistical control requires that fairly large numbers of people be studied, and that it necessitates intricate computations for which computer facilities are required as well as statistically trained personnel and time for analysis.

It is therefore not surprising that many evaluations tend to resort to quasi-experimental designs since these are, at first sight, relatively easy to work with, while the ensuing calculations appear less complicated. The methodology of quasi-experimental designs has made considerable progress over the last few decades, particularly with the growing interest in evaluation and social experiments. In fact, recent advances are so sophisticated that some quasi-experimental designs are more complex and more costly than true experimental designs (Saxe & Fine, 1981). Nevertheless, the weakness of quasi-experimental designs remains the possible selection of non-equivalent comparison groups. By selecting for comparison groups of people who differ in exposure to treatment but who may also differ in other respects, such as motivation, education, income, age, health etc., virtually any determinant of nutrition behaviour or nutritional status can be artificially introduced, thereby confounding the results. Other authors have expounded the many factors that may influence nutrition behaviour and nutritional status (Alleyne et al., 1977; Habicht & Butz, 1979; Schofield, 1979; Zeitlin, 1981). Non-treatment variables can range from macro-factors such as ecological and cultural differences between communities, meso-factors that mainly concern differences between households within communities, and micro-factors concerned with variation within households. A brief discussion of these different factors and how evaluation studies usually attempt to deal with them, follows below. (See also Box B.)

A first group of macro-factors are the variables that affect the food supply and the nutrition of communities as a whole. Examples are differences in ecology and agricultural systems, and cultural

Box B. **Sources of non-treatment variables**

The discussion in the text concentrates on confounding variables that are introduced through the use of non-equivalent comparison groups. There are two further sources of non-treatment variables that usually receive less attention:

Variables accompanying treatment

Although evaluation usually concentrates on the impact of one particular programme, it is quite possible that the programme is not the sole intervention. For example, it is not uncommon for programme staff to give medical care to children in very poor condition or to refer such cases to nearby medical personnel. An even more complex situation arises when mothers take advantage of their regular visits to a nutrition centre to visit other health facilities nearby. In such cases it is hard to decide which services can be credited with possible improvements.

Variables accompanying evaluation

Another source of confounding variables is, paradoxically, the evaluation itself, in particular when knowledge and attitude questionnaires are used on more than one occasion. Respondents often show 'habituation' effects: familiarity with the questionnaire that in itself already results in improvement in scores. Furthermore, the evaluation itself may carry with it attention by the research team that can interfere with the intervention that is being evaluated. This interference may consist of the intangible effects of repeated home-visits by research staff, but it may also take the form of advice and help given by research assistants of their own accord to the households concerned. Control groups not exposed to the treatment but equally often examined may serve to isolate such effects. Another solution is not to interview anyone more than once, i.e. not to rely on repeated interviews with the same respondents.

differences in child rearing and child nutrition practices. Differences between rural and urban living circumstances also come under this heading. Such influences obviously must somehow be kept under control during evaluation. Since these variables generally do not lend themselves to quantification, and since they also tend to show little variation within a community or over time, they are often held constant. This usually means that the evaluation is limited to a particular geographical area or particular group of people, or that different subgroups are treated separately in the analysis. In this way geographical or cultural differences are effectively eliminated, and cannot therefore offer rival explanations for observed relations between treatment and outcome.

A second group of macro-variables shows more fluctuations in time and space but still operates at group level. This concerns, for instance, seasonality or differences in access to amenities such as water supply and medical services. Seasonal variations are sometimes neutralized by carrying out studies over a short period of time, although for logistical reasons this is not always possible. Alternatively the examination of different comparison groups must be spaced equally over time, so that not one group is examined during one season, and another group during another season. Variables such as differences in the kind of water supply and access to medical services are usually handled by drawing comparison groups from the same or from similar geographical areas.

Meso-factors consist of variables affecting inter-household differences, mostly economic resources and family composition as well as a number of individual characteristics. The first comprise differences in farm size, in employment and income, in housing and sanitation, in marital arrangements, domestic stage, family size and spacing between children among others. Individual characteristics include education, motivation, health and age of parents as well as pregnancy and lactation of mothers. Again, one way of dealing with this kind of variable is to draw comparison groups from similar geographical areas with similar social and economic characteristics.

Experience has shown, however, that comparison between different areas may occasionally result in spurious differences due to influences affecting entire villages or regions (Habicht & Butz, 1979; Beaton, 1982). Moreover, the intervention is often influenced by incidental or isolated factors such as a particularly motivated assistant or co-operative village leader, which can substantially

21

contribute to success, but which can at the same time distort comparisons between villages. Furthermore, although geographical comparison can exclude individual and household variables as rival explanations for observed effects, this does not mean that they have been eliminated as sources of variation – variations that can result in corresponding variations in nutrition behaviour and nutritional status, and which can easily obscure any minor effects of intervention.

In an attempt to reduce variance as well, matching procedures are sometimes used, whereby for each individual case one or more comparison cases are selected which are identical as far as major non-treatment characteristics are concerned. A special type of matching procedure is the use of siblings as a comparison group, which is indeed effective for keeping most of the aforementioned variables under control. A disadvantage of this procedure is that siblings nearly always differ in age and that it is difficult to give them different treatments. Matching, moreover, reduces not only the variance of the non-treatment variables but that of the outcome variables as well, which results in various statistical restrictions and complications. Furthermore, only a few variables can be controlled in this way, since it is often impossible to find sufficient cases with proper matching characteristics. Finally, individual characteristics such as motivation, attitudes and personal competence are difficult to handle in this way.

Micro-factors, finally, often prove even more difficult to control. Two groups of micro-factors can be distinguished. The first concerns intra-household differences in food and nutrition: variables affecting the quantity and quality of food consumed by individual family members, together with other variables that cause differences in nutritional status between members of the same household. These variables have only recently attracted the attention of researchers, and our knowledge about them is small (Wenlock, 1980; Schofield, 1979). The second group concerns infections and other diseases, and genetic differences between children. It is usual to eliminate from evaluation any severely handicapped children and children suffering from chronic diseases, but apart from this it must be admitted that these micro-factors are usually quite difficult to control, not least because any attempt at control requires comprehensive medical examinations, which are not feasible in most studies.

Evaluations of nutrition programmes in developing countries

are often severely limited in their choice of research strategy. The daily organization of the programmes often imposes certain research designs which may be less than optimal and which do not permit the complete avoidance of the various aforementioned factors. The objective of quasi-experimental designs, however, is not so much to guard against every possible source of error, but rather to control those sources of error likely to emerge in a given situation (Weiss, 1972). It is difficult enough to realize even this limited aim. It requires knowledge about the factors that are locally important in deciding nutrition behaviour and nutritional status and it also requires knowledge about the variables that can be introduced by the selection of particular comparison groups. In most evaluations, only little prior knowledge concerning local conditions is available and although it may be possible to formulate certain broad categories of relevant variables, the exact operationalization in terms of specific factors is often not possible at the outset. By including a sufficiently large number of non-treatment variables in the data collection, the study gains a measure of flexibility which enables ad hoc operationalization of these factors. However, the refinement of non-treatment variables at a later stage, i.e. during data-analysis, is easily confounded with the evaluation as such. It is therefore necessary to use the data on a clearly delimited sub-group, such as a control group, in order to keep these calculations separate from the actual impact analysis.

In any case, when quasi-experimental designs are used sufficient information must be collected about the distribution of relevant non-treatment variables in the different groups and this information must be reported. A clear insight should be provided into the degree to which the selected design was realized as well as into any deviations from the design that have occurred. Deviations from the intended design do not necessarily invalidate results, as is often assumed. As long as sufficient information on non-treatment variables is presented, it may still be possible to take possible differences between comparison groups into account. In general, the net of evaluation should be cast widely to ensure that the role of the social environment, to which intervention and recipients belong, can be taken into proper consideration.

2.4 Nutrition Intervention Research Project (NIRP)

The Nutrition Intervention Research Project had several objectives. The first was to evaluate the impact of the three major nutrition interventions in Kenya targeted at young children: the Nutrition Field Workers; Pre-School Health Programme and Family Life Training Centres. A second objective was to study the role of differences in ecological, economic and social conditions in child nutrition and how they, in turn, relate to programme impact. Programme locations were selected in three different ecological zones in Central Province, representing some of the variations in conditions under which most of the rural population in Kenya lives and works. A third aim was to generate detailed information on child nutrition in Central Province, one of the most populous regions of Kenya, and inhabited by one of the major ethnic groups, the Kikuyu.

The three programmes were selected because they had a nationwide coverage, were well established and had been operational in Central Province for several years. Consequently the evaluation had to be adapted to the daily schedule of operations at the various centres resulting in different quasi-experimental designs. The study of the Nutrition Field Workers at MCH centres (MCH-study) was based on a comparison between selected groups of frequent and infrequent visitors; the evaluation of the Pre-School Health Programme (PSH-study) on a comparison between recent and long-time participants. At the Family Life Training centres (FLT-study) the same group of mothers[2] was interviewed at different times. Wherever possible, identical measures were used in the three studies, covering nutritional cognition, nutrition behaviour and nutritional status. The respective indicators included a questionnaire on nutritional knowledge, a scale on food preferences for young children, a dietary recall to inquire after food consumption, as well as anthropometry of young children.

Within each programme, different programme sites were selected for study. The programme sites were located in three areas at different altitudes on the slopes of the mountains that dominate the region. These areas (referred to as 'study areas') were situated near Mwea in Kirinyaga District, near Kandara in Murang'a District, and near Limuru in Kiambu District (Map 1). Mwea lies in a semi-arid area in the lower plains, Kandara is a more fertile area in the coffee

Map 1. Central Province

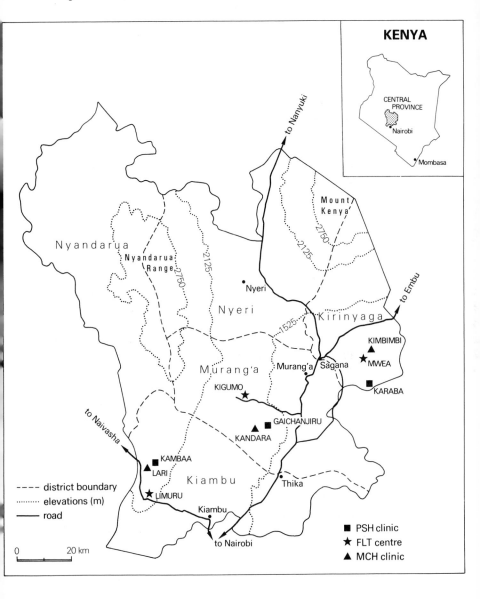

belt, while Limuru is an area at high altitude with a high agricultural potential. At the time, Central Province was the only province with three Family Life Training Centres: Kiambu FLTC (also known as Kirathimo) situated near Limuru town, Murang'a FLTC located in the administrative centre Kigumo, and Kirinyaga FLTC situated on the perimeter of the Mwea Irrigation Scheme in Wamumu. The following rural health centres were subsequently selected in the vicinity of the FLT centres: Lari, Kandara and Kimbimbi. Finally, three nearby clinics participating in the Pre-School Health Programme were selected: Kereita Mission Maternity, Gaichanjiru Mission Hospital and Karaba Mission (HN, 1980a; 1980b; 1982).

Besides the evaluation studies, the project also included some preliminary studies: the compilation of a Kikuyu dictionary of foods, meals and drinks (NIRP, 1977); a socio-economic description of the three study areas (Meilink, 1979); and studies of nutritional cognition among the Kikuyu (HN, 1978a; 1978b; 1980c).

In addition to the evaluation studies carried out in the course of 1978, a nutrition survey was conducted in Murang'a District during the same year, henceforth referred to as NIRP-survey. The primary aim of the survey was to examine the dietary patterns and nutritional status of a large group of Kikuyu children in relation to their living environment, and to furnish a reliable set of social and nutritional data for comparison purposes.[3] The detailed results of this survey have been presented in two reports (HNS, 1983; 1984); the main findings are utilized in Chapters 3 & 4 of this monograph.

The survey was carried out in two locations situated at different altitudes in Kigumo Division: 150 households in each location, 300 altogether. These two locations (referred to as survey locations) represent intermediate terrain in between the three study areas where the evaluation studies were conducted and show similar differences in ecology. The upper location, Kiiriangoro, is fertile with a high agricultural potential; the lower location, Kagurumo, is less fertile and borders the ecological zone where agricultural potential becomes marginal (Map 2).[4] The two locations differ considerably in population density, the upper having about twice the density of the lower (in 1979: 750 against 350/km^2). The population is almost exclusively Kikuyu. The year 1978 and the preceding year 1977 were both characterized by favourable weather conditions and average agricultural production.[5] In one third of

Map 2. Murang'a District

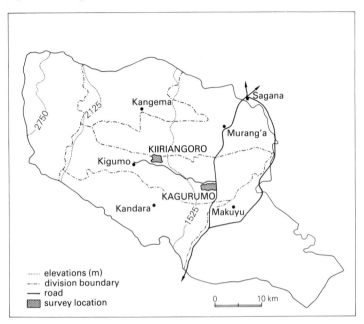

the sample, i.e. 100 households, detailed information on food consumption was collected, namely dietary records during two consecutive days, in support of the 24-hour recall data gathered in all 300 households. The same group of 100 households was further re-visited twice in the course of the following year, to serve as a control group for the evaluation at the FLT centres.

Chapter 3

Central Province & Kikuyu Society

3.1 Geography

The topography of Central Province is dominated by Mount Kenya and the Nyandarua Range. The terrain is characterized by deep valleys extending from the high grounds in the north and west, to the lower areas in the south and east. The province is divided into five districts, Nyeri and Nyandarua in the north and Kiambu, Murang'a and Kirinyaga in the east and south. As elsewhere in Central Kenya there are two distinct rainy seasons: the long rains in April and May and the short rains during November, although rainfall does vary from one year to another. The high rainfall in the higher areas feeds numerous streams flowing into the Tana and Athi rivers in the south. In the lower regions rainfall diminishes and the ridges gradually flatten out. The ridges have deeply curved flanks that consist of rich red soils, mostly humic nitosols, allowing intensive agriculture. Most of the land was formerly forested, but population increase, settlement and subsequent cultivation has resulted in the felling of much of the forest.

The agro-ecological conditions of the province are varied, ranging from upper highland to lower midland regions. Until recently the classification of agro-ecological zones in Kenya was commonly based on altitude and rainfall characteristics, and in the case of Central Province four zones were distinguished (Atlas of Kenya, 1970; Ojany & Ogendo, 1973).[1] The large majority of the population in the province, however, lives in three zones: zone II at higher altitude with pyrethrum and tea as main cash crops, zone III with coffee as the main cash crop and zone IV of a semi-arid nature and of marginal agricultural potential. Recently Jaetzold & Schmidt (1983) have composed a more detailed agro-ecological classification in which the respective zones are named after the most characteristic crops. The upper highland regions in Central Province are thus subdivided into forest zone, sheep–dairy zone and pyrethrum–wheat zone. The lower highland areas are subdivided into tea–dairy, wheat–maize–pyrethrum, and wheat–barley zones. The upper midland region comprises the coffee–tea zone, main and marginal coffee zones, sunflower–maize, and sisal zones. Finally, at the lower altitudes in Central Province there is a midland region, mainly consisting of cotton and marginal cotton zones.

The three study areas are situated at different altitudes in areas with different agro-ecological conditions (Meilink, 1979). The Limuru study area lies within Limuru Division on the southern slopes of the Nyandarua range at an altitude of over 2300m. It extends from Limuru town to Lari and Kambaa, 15km further north (Map 1). The area has a steep altitude gradient and a corresponding increase in rainfall, varying locally from 1200 to 1600mm annually, but usually being over 1400mm. The area has rich soils and a high agricultural potential. The main food crops are maize, beans and potatoes. Due to the high altitude most food crops can only be harvested once a year. Important cash crops are wattle and pyrethrum, together with horticultural and dairy products. Tea and coffee are not grown.

The Kandara study area is situated on the easterly mid-slopes of the Nyandarua range and extends from Kandara village through Gaichanjiru to Kigumo, 20km away, with altitudes ranging between 1500 and 1700m. This is land with variable vegetation and good agricultural potential with rich, fertile soils and average annual rainfall between 1400 and 1600mm, although the reliability of the first rains is less than in the Limuru area (Jaetzold & Schmidt, 1983). The area lies in the main coffee growing belt. Major food crops are maize, beans and Irish potatoes interplanted with bananas. Maize and other food crops can be harvested twice a year.

Finally, the Mwea study area lies on the southern, lower slopes of Mount Kenya in Kirinyaga District. This area extends from the villages of Karaba to Kimbimbi, 15km away along the tarmac road through the area. Altitudes range between 1100 and 1200m with rainfall of 900mm or less. This area used to be classified as semi-arid, with soils less fertile than the two other study areas and of low agricultural potential. There are, however, good possibilities for irrigated agriculture, and the Mwea–Tebere rice irrigation scheme – one of the first large-scale irrigation schemes in the country – has a dominating presence in the area. Outside the scheme drought-resistant grains and roots are grown as the main food crops; cash crops are cotton and grams.

3.2 Population

In 1979 the population of Central Province numbered 2.3 million, about 15% of Kenya's total population. Population density for the total province is 178 (only Western and Nyanza Provinces have higher figures). Within the province there are variations in population patterns between districts as well as ecological zones. The highest population concentration is found in Kiambu District (280), reflecting the nearby presence of the Nairobi agglomeration. Next highest densities are in the ancestral districts of Murang'a (261) and Kirinyaga (202); Nyeri (148) and Nyandarua (66) were settled later in history. More important than the differences in population density between districts are the differences between different ecological zones. Areas above the forest line are largely uninhabited. The highland and midland zones covering about half the provincial territory, have a high agricultural potential and form a densely populated belt running through the province. Here population densities average between 400 and 500, and in some areas reach 700 or more. The lower zones are less fertile and form a less hospitable environment with far fewer people: around 100–200/km². The three study areas differ accordingly and the population densities were estimated to have been as follows at the time of the 1969 census: Limuru 410; Kandara 390 and Mwea 110/km². At the time of the next census in 1979 these were 454, 552 and 140 respectively.[2] It is evident that with a predominantly rural population and a national population growth of nearly 4%, the problems of land scarcity and subdivision of plots will be aggravated in the near future. The population consists almost exclusively of Kikuyu, particularly in the rural areas where more than 95% of the people are of Kikuyu origin. The Kikuyu belong to the North-East Bantu-speaking peoples. They migrated southwards along Mount Kenya in the fifteenth and sixteenth centuries, subsequently dispersing through Murang'a and later towards Nyeri to the north and Kiambu to the south (Muriuki, 1974). The first contacts with Europeans and colonial rule date from the end of the nineteenth century. At that time the Kikuyu numbered some 500,000 people, organized in a system of age groups and lineages. Age groups and membership of the extended family were an important source of identity for the individual. Political decision making and landownership were vested in the lineages. There were no chiefs in this largely egalitarian society, and only limited social stratification (Middleton & Kershaw, 1965; Leakey, 1977).

Kikuyu society has undergone dramatic changes since the beginning of this century. The age group system was soon discontinued and the nuclear family became increasingly important. The most turbulent period in recent history was the Mau-Mau struggle for independence (Buijtenhuijs, 1971). There has been a shift towards individual landownership culminating in the land consolidation between 1955 and 1965. Social stratification has become more prominent and is now an important factor in rural Kikuyu society. The reasons and mechanisms underlying this transformation have been described by Tignor (1976); land reform has been studied by Sorrenson (1967). Contemporary daily life of the Kikuyu must be viewed against the background of these profound social changes.

The rest of this chapter is devoted to a discussion of the main economic and domestic characteristics underlying present-day Kikuyu society. Kikuyu food culture and child nutrition are discussed in Chapter 4. In both chapters data from the NIRP-survey as well as published data from other sources have been used.

3.3 Rural Economy: Agriculture & Wage Employment

As in the rest of Kenya, agriculture is the mainstay of the rural economy: smallholder farms and large estates. Large coffee estates are situated in the southern part of Kiambu District. Sisal and pineapple plantations are found in the lower, eastern part of Kiambu and Murang'a District. The estate sector, however, is surpassed by the smallholder sector in terms of area cultivated and agricultural output and even more in terms of the number of people dependent on it. Since Independence there has been an impressive growth of smallholder farm production, both in respect of commercial crops and food crops (Meilink, 1979).

Agricultural land is divided into holdings, the plots of land as registered at the land office. Many holdings are occupied by more than one household and the most common situation is land shared between patrilineally related households, such as land divided between a father and his sons or, after the father's death, between his sons. However, more than one quarter of the households do not share the holding with other households and live independently. This is more often the case in the lower, less densely populated areas. In the upper areas holdings are more often subdivided and when shared also divided into more sub-plots (HNS, 1983: 26). Even when land is shared, households are usually independent of each other; each having its own kitchen and working its own part of the land (Box C). The nationwide Integrated Rural Survey[3] of 1978 counted 500,000 rural households in Central Province (CBS, 1981a). Many households do not own a farm or operate relatively small farms: nearly one quarter were classified as not operating any farmland, and another quarter as having less than one acre at their disposal. In this respect the situation in Central Province resembles the rest of rural Kenya (Table 1). Only a minority of

Table 1. *Smallholder farm size (1978) (hectares)*

	Central Province (%)	Kenya (%)
None	22	22
0.01–0.4	28	25
0.5–0.9	20	20
1.0–1.9	15	16
2.0 and more	16	17

Source: CBS, 1981a: 89

Box C. **Division of land**

The division of land between fathers and sons and later between heirs is a complex process. One aim of the land consolidation carried out in Central Province between 1955 and 1965 was to prevent fragmentation of land and at the time when consolidation was completed further division of smallholdings was prohibited (Sorrenson, 1967), although this has not stopped further fragmentation. During the past century there has been a decisive shift from communal towards individual landownership; land consolidation in fact putting the final seal on this development. This, if anything, made sons even more dependent upon their fathers than before.

Land may be divided temporarily or permanently. In the first case, the land is divided at the start of each season, in the second case each household uses certain parts of the land permanently, although nothing is really permanent in this regard (Maas, 1986). The type of division has to do with several factors. Firstly, the age of the married children: a young couple may have to wait one or two seasons before getting some land. This depends on, among other things, whether the young husband is resident or works elsewhere. In the latter case his wife may have to wait a bit longer. Secondly, a related factor is whether people have invested in the farm. Coffee seedlings are expensive and take five years to mature and produce the first harvest; such an investment requires permanent control of the land concerned.

Over the years, however, divisions of land tend to become more formal and in the end there is usually a permanent division between the father and his sons. Sons who reside elsewhere with their families may or may not be allocated their part of the land at this time but they will certainly claim their rights when the father dies. This does not mean that all sons will receive equal shares; differences in opportunities elsewhere and education received during the lifetime of the father often are taken into account, while elder sons may receive larger plots than their younger brothers. In exceptional circumstances single or separated daughters may be allocated a piece of land but usually they work on the sub-plot which the parents have reserved for themselves.

households (30%) have farms that are larger than 1ha (2.5 acres). Earlier on, 3 acres was considered the minimum farm size necessary to assure the livelihood of an average household.[4] Ecological conditions, the quality of the land and other farming conditions, strongly influence farm size. Although variations in soil fertility occur within ecological zones, the differences between ecological zones are generally more pronounced, and in the lower areas farm sizes generally tend to be larger. Because of this, the actual size of the farm says little about the resources of individual households. Much more important in determining the level of resources of individual households is the use that is made of available land.

Of the areas cultivated in Central Province, 20–25% is reserved for commercial crops, the remaining 75% for different food crops (Table 2). Of the total food production, about two thirds was used for subsistence purposes, the remaining one third for sales. This

Table 2. *Smallholder cultivation in Central Province (1978)*

	Central Province	*Kenya*
Area cultivated ('000ha)	*291*	*2046*
Food crops	73%	89%
Commercial crops	27%	11%
Food crop production[1] (million bags)	*12.85*	*32.5*
Subsistence purposes	65%	85%
Commercial purposes	35%	15%

[1] Estimates based on production figures for maize, beans, and English potatoes
Source: CBS, 1981a: 111, 112, 113, 118, 120

means that about half of the agricultural activity in Central Province is commercial, which is much more than in the rest of Kenya. It is not surprising that a large proportion of the inputs used nationally in the smallholder sector are channelled to Central Province (nearly 60% of the fertilizer and sprays) (CBS, 1981a: 108).

Nearly all households that have farmland grow food crops, land and farming conditions permitting. Most of the households with farmland grow maize and about half the smallholders grow beans (CBS, 1981a: 111, 112). Many people grow bananas, various roots and tubers; the majority of households also grow vegetables. The possibilities for cultivation of different food crops vary with ecological conditions, as mentioned earlier.[5] Many households keep livestock: one or more cows (45% of the households), goats (25%), sheep (30%), and chickens (55%) (CBS, 1981: 96–102). Goats and sheep are commonly kept for traditional purposes, such as exchange or slaughter at festivities and ceremonial occasions. They are also sold at local markets for immediate cash purposes. Smallholder milk production in Central Province is much higher than in the rest of Kenya (with the exception of Rift Valley Province): an average of 500 litres per household annually. Of the milk produced, one third is sold to neighbours or to buying organizations, notably dairy co-operatives and the Kenya Cooperative Creameries (CBS, 1981a: 95). The remainder is used at home. Eggs are also sold but mainly to neighbours and at local markets.

The major crops grown for commercial purposes are coffee and tea, cultivated by 20% and 17% of the smallholders respectively (CBS, 1981a: 120). Since these figures are provincial averages the proportion of farmers in the zones suitable for these crops is much higher. The next crop in order of commercial importance is vegetables, the production of which has increased greatly in recent years. A considerable number of farmers cultivate specialized crops such as cucumbers and tomatoes, or vegetable seedlings for the local market. In some households commercial farming is a well-planned activity, in others commercial farming is of marginal significance: when in need of money they sell some of their food stock at the local market. Most of the commercial farming is agricultural in nature, but there is also livestock rearing. Some households concentrate on a single activity or crop, others engage in several activities and different crops. Because of this variety in practices it is not easy to distinguish the degree of commercial farming of individual households. The Integrated Rural Survey made a distinction between households that operate their farms primarily to grow food for the family, and households that produce for household consumption as well as (or mainly) for sales. Nationally, 38% of the farming households belong to this second category; in Central Province this is 40% (CBS, 1981a: 87). The NIRP-survey used a more detailed classification procedure (see section 3.6) and, in these survey locations, 33% of the households were substantially involved in commercial farming. The remaining group is involved mostly in subsistence farming,[6] although such terminology suggests an absolute difference while the difference is, of course, only one of degree. Commercial farmers also grow food for their own consumption, while the non-commercial farmers usually sell some of their produce as well.

The NIRP-survey also found that the extent of commercial farming is not different in ecological zones, provided that allowance is made for different commercial activities. In the upper ecological zones, coffee and tea cultivation are the most important activity, while production in the lower areas is more diversified, with more farmers selling food crops and keeping livestock and poultry for sales.[7]

In the rural areas of Central Province many men, and certainly most of the married men, engage in gainful activity outside their farm (CBS, 1981a: 49). According to the Integrated Rural Survey, 45% of the heads of households had their main occupation outside their own holding. In other areas of Kenya this percentage is much lower, i.e. between 20% and 30%. The remaining group is not without off-farm income, because many men participate in casual or day-labour. Indeed, the NIRP-survey found that 35% of the husbands had regular employment with government or industry and 17% were self-employed as traders, artisans or shopkeepers, but that another 35% were engaged in day-labour of various kinds. Because employment opportunities in the rural areas are limited, up to 50% of the husbands are (temporarily) resident elsewhere. The absences from home are, however, not prolonged like those of migrant labourers elsewhere in Kenya because Nairobi, the main job market, is relatively near. Some husbands commute weekly or even more often, others stay away for longer periods. Most husbands, however, visit their homes quite regularly, at least once every fortnight (HNS, 1983: 37).

Many of the self-employed men held regular jobs in the past, providing them with the financial means to start their private enterprises. The income of the self-employed and regularly employed is generally higher than that of day-labourers, whose income is not only uncertain but whose wages are low. Even when day-labourers work in the urban areas where wages tend to be higher, the extra income is quickly lost to the expense of living in town, and little money remains to be taken home (Box D).

The labour of women is firstly directed at the home and the farm. According to the traditional division of farm labour between

Box D. **Husbands and wages**

It is sometimes alleged that husbands are largely to blame for the malnutrition occurring among Kikuyu children. The argument is based on the assumption that men generally take the best parts of the daily dishes and that at the same time they squander the household income on drink and girlfriends (Stamp, 1975). The findings of the NIRP-survey, however, did not support this. The financial contribution of the husband to household expenditure is firstly decided by the type of occupation (Figure 1). Nearly all husbands with regular employment paid the expenses for children's clothes but they also contributed to daily household expenses. The contribution to household expenses is the first to decrease with lesser income from wage employment, but most husbands without regular employment still try to pay for the children's clothes, one of the first financial responsibilities of a Kikuyu husband.

Figure 1. *Husbands paying for household expenses and children's clothing*

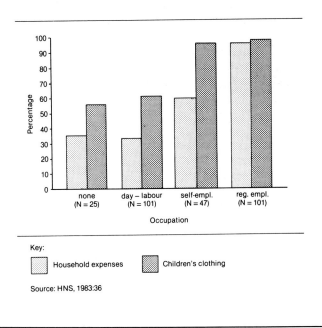

Key:

Household expenses   Children's clothing

Source: HNS, 1983:36

men and women, the husbands are responsible for breaking new land, cultivating cash crops and looking after cattle. Wives are responsible for the cultivation of food crops and domestic chores. With so many husbands living away from home this division is by now more nominal than real. Many women are in charge of all farming activities, if not wholly responsible for the farm, although there is considerable variation between households in this respect. Consequently women spend a lot of time and labour on the cultivation of cash crops, a trend which is far more pronounced here than elsewhere in Kenya. In Central Province more women than men are regularly occupied with the planting, weeding and harvesting of the food crops (90% against 40%), the same being the case with the commercial crops such as coffee (30% against 20%).[8] The sale of cash crops, however, is still organized in the usual way, which means that the earnings of commercial farming are handled by the husband. The women do have control over the proceeds from the sale of food crops and from the trading activities they engage in. However, the actual arrangements differ from family to family; in some cases women trade in their husband's name which means that they have to account for the money earned (Box E).

There are very few opportunities for regular employment for rural housewives and the only possibility of earning wages is casual labour[9] with neighbours or at estates that usually lie further away. Day-labour carries a low status (particularly when the employer is a wealthy neighbour) and points to a lack of other resources in the household. Women who have little land available and who do not receive an adequate income from their husbands are inevitably dependent on it for the upkeep of their family. Women from other households can also engage in day-labour, but less frequently and usually at harvest-time, when wages are higher. If the husband is regularly employed and if the household farms commercially, the housewife seldom engages in day-labour because she often acts as a kind of farm manager and has no time to spare.

Different estimates place the percentage of households in Central Province below the poverty line at around 20% which is less than the national average (Table 3). Greer and Thorbecke (1983), taking regional differences in existing diets into account, arrive at an estimate of 33% of the households in Central Province below the food poverty line of 2250kcal. per consumption unit. The NIRP-survey demonstrated that the 40% of households that were

---

***Box E.* Domestic workload**

The workload of women apart from work on the farm and any wage employment, of course, consists firstly of domestic chores such as cooking, cleaning, washing, looking after children, mending clothes etc. Physically probably most demanding are collecting firewood and fetching water. Most people still draw water from the river, which means a regular walk uphill with a full container. In the majority of households water is collected two or three times a day, often by the housewife herself but also by children who are strong enough to carry the weight. The vast majority of households use firewood but this is acquired in different ways. In the less densely populated areas nearly all women collect firewood on their own farm or in the neighbourhood. In the more densely settled areas only a minority of women can collect firewood from their own farm while the others who are not so lucky and cannot collect in the neighbourhood have to buy firewood from elsewhere, often at a considerable distance from the home.

In many households women receive some assistance with their household chores although this is closely connected with the domestic (life) stage of the family. Most help comes from elder children. Many mothers-in-law live quite near, even in the same compound, but only few lend a helping hand. Not surprising, since it is the younger woman who should help her mother-in-law according to Kikuyu custom. Husbands also rarely assist with daily household tasks. As many as half the mothers of young children seem not to receive any help with their household work. In case of illness and other emergencies, however, many husbands as well as mothers-in-law do look after the children (HNS, 1983: 41).

---

qualified as poor[10] not only had a smaller share in the money economy but also had less potential for self-subsistence and that their food situation is probably precarious (Table 4). Of the rich households approximately 75% reported that they are able to grow enough food for their own consumption, of the medium households about 40%, and very few of the poor households (25%). The same applies to the number of households that have milk or eggs available: the percentage drops from 80% in rich households, to 45% or less in poor households. It is not only the households that

Table 3. *Estimates of smallholder poverty in Central Province (% households below poverty line)*

	Central Province	Kenya
Income based		
(Collier & Lal, 1980)	22	34
Consumption based		
(Livingstone, 1981)	18	39
(ILO, 1983)	19	24
(Greer & Thorbecke, 1983)	33	41

Source: CBS/UNICEF, 1984: 57–8

are able to grow enough food that sell food crops. Surprisingly, in the NIRP-survey, of the households reporting insufficient food production to meet their own demands, 17% nevertheless did sell foods occasionally.

3.4 Residential Characteristics

The residential pattern of Kikuyu in the rural areas is patri- or neo-local. Sons marry and settle on the land of their fathers or acquire land elsewhere to strike out on their own, while daughters, upon marriage, leave home to follow their husbands. Usually,

Table 4. *Food availability in different income groups (%)*

	Income group		
	Poor (N=123)	Medium (N=114)	Rich (N=63)
Food crops (Reportedly able to grow *enough* food to feed members household)	25	44	76
Milk (Available from home production)	32	54	80
Eggs (Available from home production)	45	61	85

Source: NIRP-survey (HNS, 1983: 32)

sons build their houses next to that of their father. Sometimes a second compound is built elsewhere on the holding because of the terrain or because of quarrels between households. Around the houses a small area is cleared where most day-time activities take place.

Traditionally, married women lived with their children in one hut, the husband having a separate hut while teenage sons would build a so-called 'boys' house'. Nowadays husbands no longer have a separate hut, although a small house or room with a separate entrance is still built for the grown-up boys in as many as half the cases. When no boys' house is available in the compound, sleeping arrangements for grown-up boys are sometimes made with their peers in neighbouring compounds; they are not supposed to sleep with their parents under the same roof. Traditionally, huts were built from wooden poles and planks with a thatched roof and a kitchen in the centre (Andersen, 1977). Nowadays most houses are rectangular buildings with corrugated iron roofs and comprise several rooms. Since suitable wood is scarce and expensive, walls today are usually made of mud on a frame of pole and twines. A small number of houses have stone walls and/or paved floors. The Integrated Rural Survey reported the following housing characteristics: roof (corrugated iron 57%, thatched 32%); walls (mud 71%, wood 15%, stone 12%); floors (earth 87%, concrete 11%) (CBS, 1981a: 634). In small houses the kitchen is often combined with the living room but in larger houses it is usually a separate room or even a separate building (Sterkenburg, 1978).

The kitchen usually contains no more than the minimum necessities for cooking: a container to collect water, a few gourds, some stools and perhaps a small cupboard. Cheap crockery and cutlery have replaced the traditional implements; instead of earthen pots most housewives now use *sufuria's*, the grey, aluminium vessels without a lid that are found all over East Africa, although for some dishes earthenware is still preferred. Most housewives in the rural areas still prepare meals over a wood fire as their grandmothers used to do, wedging pots and pans between three big stones. Some families also use a charcoal stove or *jiko*. Paraffin lamps are the source of lighting in more than three-quarters of the households (CBS, 1981a: 63, 84). Around 60% of the households get their water from a stream, 15% from a spring, well or piped supply, and the remaining 25% from another source. The average distance to the water source in the dry season is about 0.9km.

Sanitation usually consists of a pit latrine; 90% of the households in Central Province have this means of sewage disposal, which is an uncommonly high percentage by Kenyan standards (CBS, 1981a: 66–68).

3.5 Domestic Characteristics

The average age at first marriage of women in Central Province is 19 years, which is somewhat later than the national average. The fertility of young women in Central Province therefore remains slightly behind the national rate, but over the age of 25, fertility rates are equal to or slightly above the national average. The present generation of women over 45 has, on average, given birth to eight children (CBS, 1980).

The average household size in Central Province is 5.1 and the typical household consists of the nuclear family: man, wife and children. More than 70% of the households count seven members or less (CBS, 1981a: 92). Some households have an occasional relative living with them, and some can be said to consist of extended families spanning more than one generation. However, there are very few households with such large numbers: only 6% of the households consist of eleven or more persons. About 30% of the households are female-headed and this group includes a variety of family situations: widows, unmarried women with children, and households where the husband works elsewhere and no longer visits frequently without however officially separating. Single women generally live with their parents, also when they have given birth to one or more children. Separated and divorced women often attempt to return to the parental homestead or move in with a married brother. In the rural areas the number of separated women is small, despite the fact that 11% of the first marriages of Kikuyu women are reportedly dissolved within the first ten years (CBS, 1980: 79).[11] There is little room for separated women in rural society. As long as a woman lives on her husband's land or on that of her in-laws she is considered married, whatever the further state of matrimony. Once a woman leaves her husband and returns to her parents she is rarely given a warm welcome because the land rightfully belongs to her brothers, and often considerable pressure is put on her to return to her husband. Alternatively she can try to find another husband as soon as possible. Often she has no choice but to find an existence elsewhere, for example in town or as a labourer at the coffee and tea estates. There is a low incidence of polygamy. About 7.5% of the married women live in polygamous unions, about 10% of the married men, one of the lowest rates in Kenya (CBS, 1980). Traditionally, the wives of one husband lived in separate houses in the same compound but nowadays they usually live in different places.

The striking thing about present-day Kikuyu life is the degree to which the nuclear family predominates. Relatively few households have a composition other than husband, wife and children, although many husbands reside elsewhere for reasons of employment. Variations in family composition occur mainly in respect of domestic stage (described below) and the number of children in different age groups.

A young Kikuyu couple needs time to settle in. The young wife usually moves to her husband's compound and she has to adapt to her new family relations, in particular to her mother-in-law. This settling in, though, implies more than getting to know new people. The recently married often have to wait some time before they are allocated land by the husband's father (Box C, p. 33). The birth of the first child is an important occasion because it gives proof of the fertility of the union. Young mothers have to learn to tend their babies. Some are good at it but others are less gifted or less dedicated, and this does not escape the notice of the mother-in-law. Gradually after the birth of more children, when it appears that the children will survive and the marriage will last, the young woman will establish a position among the other women of the family. The duration of this early period in the domestic cycle differs individually, but roughly it can be said to last until the first-born child reaches the age of six. This is also more or less the age at which, traditionally, the child and its parents would have gone through the important second-birth ceremony (Leakey, 1977: 550); nowadays it is about the age when the child starts attending primary school.

Families then enter a 'middle-stage' period which may last for some ten years, and in which they generally consolidate their position. With school-going and pre-school children present, families increase in size until they reach their final or near-final number. Since, as noted, nearly all families with young children consist of man, wife and children, variations in family size mainly concern the number of children. However, the number of children as such is not as important in deciding family dynamics as their age composition, i.e. the number of children in different age groups. Young children make the greatest demands on the attention of the mother, although Kikuyu children soon learn to look after themselves. By the age of six or earlier they start to do small jobs, notably looking after the very youngest children. When physically stronger they have to carry water, collect firewood and generally help on the farm after school hours, the girls more so than the boys. Gradually children relieve the mother of some of her workload. Once they reach the age of 17 they are regarded as grown-up and are expected to contribute their labour to the household either as wage earners or as help with household and farm duties. This also indicates the next step in the domestic cycle, what may be termed the 'senior' family stage. Traditionally, this step was the circumcision of the first-born child which for girls usually took place between the ages of 10 and 14 years and for boys between 15 and 18 years. This was an important occasion not only for the child but also for its parents, because it marked their acceptance among the elders of the tribe (Leakey, 1977c: 996). In the present day such formal rites of passage for the parents have largely disappeared. Nevertheless, the time when the first-born child reaches the age of 16–17 and comes to be regarded as an adult is still an important transition. Further domestic stages can similarly be distinguished, for example, when the eldest child marries and when there are no longer any younger children in the family. These later stages, however, are of less relevance in the context of the nutrition of young children.

3.6 Social–Economic Differentiation

On the basis of the previous discussion three important factors can be identified that distinguish between Kikuyu households and that are potentially important in deciding the nutrition of young children: income group, domestic stage and the number of children in the youngest age group. As will be shown below on the basis of the NIRP-survey data, domestic stage and income group combine many individual variables, while the number of young children represents an additional aspect of family life. The division into income groups reflects the degree of involvement of households in the money economy. It is based on the extent of commercial farming, on the one hand, and the type of off-farm employment of the husband on the other hand. Commercial farming is defined as substantial involvement in one specific commercial activity, i.e. when half an acre is under cash crop cultivation or if food crops are sold regularly. Also included among the commercial farmers are households that are involved simultaneously in two or more minor activities[12] and the households that reportedly employ farm labour.[13] As regards income from employment, husbands (and households) can be distinguished into regularly employed (with government or industry, including the self-employed) and the not regularly employed (including day labourers and those not working outside their farm[14]). Some households are in the favourable position where husbands have regular employment and where households also farm commercially. These households are generally well-off and, by rural standards, can be qualified as 'rich'. At the other end of the scale there is a large group of households that are not in a position to farm commercially and where husbands have no regular employment either. By the same standards these can be regarded as 'poor' households. In between are households with one major source of income, either regular employment or commercial farming, here referred to as the 'medium' income group. This threefold classification into income groups makes it possible to sidestep the problems inherent in estimating household incomes in money terms, which would be particularly difficult and unreliable in this case, with so many husbands being non-resident. On the basis of this classification about 40% of the households in the NIRP-survey were classified as poor, another 40% as belonging to a medium income group and 20% as belonging to rich households.[15]

There are all kinds of related differences between income groups that confirm the validity of this classification (Table 5). The rich households are more likely to live in houses built of wood or stone,[16] to have a water tank on the premises and sometimes even to use an energy source other than firewood. These are obvious indicators of social status and limited mainly to the rich households. The women who engage in day-labour are mainly from poor households. In fact, a few women from rich households employ domestic servants themselves. Women from this income group are generally more educated than women from medium and poor households. Although the division into income groups is not based on farm size as such (intentionally because the classification was meant to cut across ecological variations of soil and climate), farm size does, of course, play a part: the average farm size of

Table 5. *Characteristics of households in different income groups*

	Income group		
	Poor (N=123)	Medium (N=114)	Rich (N=63)
Farm size (average, acres)	1.7	2.4	3.7
Residence, husband (% elsewhere)	25	72	63
Education, mother (% Standard 5 or more)	23	38	57
Employment (% mother engages in day labour)	75	48	13
House (% wooden/stone walls)	8	6	27
Water supply (% tank/tap on premises)	3	5	21
Energy source (% other than firewood)	2	1	8
Household labour (% employ household labour)	—	—	10

Source: NIRP-survey (HNS, 1983: 44)

rich households is twice that of poor households, with medium households in between.

   Three domestic stages can be distinguished among families with young children: 'young', 'middle' and 'senior' stage. The first period covers the early years of marriage when children are still young;[17] the second stage begins when the first-born child reaches the age of six years; the family arrives at the third, senior stage when the first-born child reaches the age of 17. Associated with domestic stages are other aspects of family life (Table 6). At some time in the course of subsequent domestic stages many families start to live on their own. The size of the family also increases and more people have to be looked after. For example, in senior families water has to be collected more often – to mention only one aspect of the greater workload involved. On the other hand, with time women are able to command more help in the household, assistance that is given largely by the elder children. In general, there is no relation between domestic stage and income group to which the household belongs. Whether poor or rich households, the percentage of young or senior families is roughly the same.[18] While it is true that senior families have more land to farm and more often own cattle, fewer women in senior than in young families report that they are able to grow enough food to feed the members of the household.

Table 6. *Characteristics of families at different domestic stages*

	Domestic stage		
	Young (N=75)	Middle (N=171)	Senior (N=54)
Residence (% independent)	5	24	45
Household size (average no. of people)	4.1	7.1	9.1
Water supply (% collect 3× or more per day)	25	51	59
Household help (% women reporting help from others)	35	58	85
Farm size (average, acres)	1.3	2.2	4.3
Cattle (average number)	0.6	1.0	1.3
Food availability (% reportedly able to grow enough food to feed members of household)	60	40	28

Source: NIRP-survey (HNS, 1983: 50)

In general, family size increases with domestic stage but internal family dynamics are also strongly influenced by the number of children in different age groups. The analysis in this monograph concentrates on the number of very young children in the household, distinguishing between households with few (one or two) children and households with several (three or more) children under the age of five years. Children under five require most attention of the mother, and the quality of child care she can give in addition to her other duties is probably quite directly related to the number of children of that age requiring her attention. Older children can cope better for themselves and are also less likely to suffer from less maternal attention. This third factor can therefore be seen as an important indicator of the quality of child care, and it is independent of income group[19] and largely independent of domestic stage;[20] i.e. the number of young children can vary regardless of whether a household is at a young or senior domestic stage or whether it belongs to a rich or poor income group.

In sum, important distinctions between Kikuyu households with young children – our main focus of interest – concern income group, domestic stage and number of young children. These three factors are, statistically speaking, largely independent of each other. They will be used in the rest of this monograph as the means, first of analyzing the role of economic and social conditions in child nutrition (starting in the next chapter), and second, for purposes of control in the evaluation studies.

Chapter 4

Food Culture & Child Nutrition

4.1 Foods & Dishes

The food habits of the Kikuyu have changed considerably over the past century. People used to grow a variety of grains and early in the century finger millet was still an important staple food together with sorghum (Anderson, 1937; Proctor, 1926; Orr & Gilks, 1931). Nowadays the areas under cultivation with millet and sorghum are insignificant; when needed these grains are usually purchased. They have largely been replaced by maize which was introduced early in the last century; yellow maize initially but later, in the first decades of this century, white maize became popular, and nowadays is highly preferred (Paterson, 1943; Bertin et al., 1971).

Various types of roots, tubers and starchy fruits are also grown. Irish potatoes which were introduced only at the end of the last century have become very popular; green banana and sweet potato are also grown widely. Cassava, yam and taro (locally called arrow root) are far less common.

The kidney bean is the most common legume, together with the ordinary pea and the cowpea. The Bonavist bean and the pigeon pea are regarded as delicacies and served in ceremonial dishes at

Table 7. *Foods currently used in rural areas of Central Province*[1]

ENGLISH	SCIENTIFIC	KIKUYU[2]
Cereals		
maize	zea mays	mbembe
maize flour	zea mays	mutu wa mbembe
millet, bullrush, flour	pennisetum americanum	mutu wa mwere
millet, finger, flour	eleusine coracane	mutu wa mugimbi
rice	oryza sativa	mucere
sorghum, flour	sorghum spp.	mutu wa muhia
wheat, flour	triticum vulgare	mutu wa ngano
Roots, tubers & starchy fruits		
cassava	manihot esculenta	mwanga (s); mianga (p)
green banana	musa paradisiaca	irigu (s); marigu (p)
potato, Irish	solanum tuberosum	waru
potato, sweet	ipomoea batatas	ngwaci
taro	colocasia esculenta	nduma
yam	dioscorea spp.	gikwa (s); ikwa (p)
Grain legumes		
bean, bonavist	lablab niger	njahi
bean, kidney	phaseolus vulgaris	mboco
bean, lima	phaseolus lunatus	noe
bean, mung, green	phaseolus aureus	ndengu; ngina; thuu
groundnut	arachis hypogaea	njugu karanga
pea	pisum, sativum	minji
pea, cow	vigna spp.	thoroko
pea, pigeon	cajanus cajan	njugu
Vegetables		
amaranth	amaranthus spp.	terere
cabbage; cabbage leaves	brassica oleracea	kabici
carrots	daucus carota	karati
cauliflower	brassica oleracea	kariburawa
kale	brassica oleracea	thukuma
leaves, bonavist bean		nyeni cia macahi
leaves, cassava		nyeni cia mianga
leaves, cow pea		nyeni cia mathoroko
leaves, Irish potato		nyeni cia waru
leaves, kidney bean		maboco
leaves, pumpkin		nyeni cia marenge
leaves, taro		marutu
lettuce	lactuca sativa	rethithi
onion	allium cepa	gitunguru (s); itunguru (p)
peppers, red and sweet	capsicum annuum	biribiri
pumpkin	cucurbita spp.	irenge (s); marenge (p)
spinach	spinacia oleracea	mathibinaci
tomato	lycopersicum esculentum	nyanya

Food Culture & Child Nutrition

ENGLISH	SCIENTIFIC	KIKUYU[2]
Fruits		
apple, custard	annona spp.	itomoko (s); matomoko (p)
avocado pear	persea americana	ikorobia (s); makorobia (p)
banana, sweet	musa sapientum	riru (s); meru (p)
berries	rubus spp.	ndare
cape gooseberry	physalis peruviana	nathi
grapefruit	citrus grandis	irimau (s); marimau (p)
guava	psidium guajava	ibera (s); mbera (p)
lemon	citrus aurantifolia	ndimu
mango	mangifera indica	iembe (s); maembe (p)
mulberry	morus alba	ituya (s); matuya (p)
orange	citrus sinensis	icungwa (s); macungwa (p)
passion fruit	passiflora edulis	ndunda (s); matunda (p)
paw-paw	carica papaya	ibabai (s); mababai (p)
pear	pyrus communis	ngario; mugumo(s) migumo(p)
pineapple	ananas cosmosus	inanathi (s); mananathi (p)
		riinabu (s); mainabu (p)
plum, red; yellow	prunus domestica	nduramuthi; ndarathini
tangerine	citrus reticulata	thandara
Condiments & spices		
coriander, leaves	coriandrum sativum	ndania
curry powder		mbithari
ginger powder	zingiber officinale	tangauthi
sodium bicarbonate		igata
salt		cumbi
Meats & animal products		
beef		nyama cia ng'ombe
chicken		nyama cia nguku
egg		itumbi (s); matumbi (p)
fish		thamaki
goat		nyama cia mburi
milk		iria
milk powder		iria ria mutu
mutton		nyama cia ngurwe
rabbit		nyama cia mbuku
Miscellaneous		
butter; margarine		thiagi
fat, cooking		maguta ma kuruga
ghee		thamuri
honey		uuki
sugar		cukari
sugar cane		kigwa (s); igwa (p)

[1] Originally published in *Ecology of Food and Nutrition*, 1980, 142–3.
[2] Food names in Kikuyu are listed in singular (s) and plural (p). Names that are
known in only one form are given without further indication.

marriage and childbirth. The lima bean, which is locally called soya bean, the mung bean and the groundnut are available but less frequently used. The vegetables most often prepared are kale, cabbage, pumpkin leaves and (young) cowpea leaves. The leaves of other legumes are also eaten but less often. Kale (sukuma wiki) has become very popular although introduced only recently. It has probably replaced many other plant leaves, particularly many of the wild varieties whose consumption seems to have greatly declined. Onions, peppers, tomatoes and carrots are the most frequent seasonings. Fruits are usually eaten between meals. Sweet banana, mango and passion fruit in particular are popular. Most fruits are not difficult to obtain when in season but some foods such as cape gooseberries, pears, plums and tangerines are only grown in certain areas.

A list of the foods consumed in the rural areas is given in Table 7. The list includes foods, such as fish and certain fruits, which are rarely eaten and perhaps never used in certain households. Truly exceptional items such as antelope meat, grasshoppers or stinging nettle, however, are not included.

Usually a family eats three meals a day: breakfast, a second meal early in the afternoon between 1 and 3 pm and the last meal in the evening between 7 and 9. After these meals people often drink tea prepared with plenty of milk and sugar. Tea may also be taken in the morning or afternoon. The staple food is maize, which can be roasted or boiled on the cob when fresh, but usually the grains are removed from the cob before preparation ('dry maize'). The favourite dish is maize and kidney beans boiled together (*githeri*). Sometimes peas or other types of beans may be added or may replace the kidney beans. Occasionally some meat may also be added. The ratio of maize and beans[1] shows wide variation depending on such factors as taste and availability, while young children are often given more beans or, when very young, beans only. Githeri is usually prepared in large quantities sufficient for several days. Individual meals usually consist of a portion of this basic dish to which vegetables, bananas,[1] potatoes,[1] or seasonings may be added to give some variety to the main meals of the day. When roots and tubers are added to the githeri the dish may be mashed but in some areas this is hardly ever done.

Another basic dish is a stiff porridge of maize flour (*ngima*) served either when whole maize is not available or as a quick dish that requires little time to prepare. Ngima is usually eaten with a vegetable stew consisting of fat, onions and leafy vegetables to which tomatoes and fresh beans or peas may be added when in season. It can also be taken with tea or milk. *Ucuru* is a thin porridge of maize, millet or sorghum flour. Another basic dish is *gitoero*, a stew of roots and tubers, such as Irish potatoes and green bananas.[2] More elaborate gitoero dishes can also be prepared with vegetables, meat or seasonings. Some roots like sweet potato are also eaten single, boiled in the skin. Sometimes a rice dish with gitoero or a stew may be served. *Chapatis*, unleavened bread, and pancakes are occasionally prepared. Snacks include bread, biscuit, cakes and soft drinks which are on sale at many of the local shops.

Meat consumption plays a relatively minor role. The first ethnographers already reported that meat was the luxury of the few and only eaten in small quantities on occasions of sacrifices or festivals (Routledge and Routledge, 1910). Sometimes meat is added to the family dish on special occasions, and adult men also buy roasted meat in bars and at other selling points. The meats consumed are mostly beef, mutton, goat and chicken. Children are given fairly large quantities of milk to drink, pure or diluted with water, or served with tea. Spices are largely absent from Kikuyu cooking, and limited to salt and, sometimes, curry powder. Ginger powder is sometimes added to tea, while sodium bicarbonate may occasionally be used in cooking vegetables not so much to add taste as to make the leaves more tender.

4.2 Nutritional Cognition

The Kikuyu word for food is *irio*, although in the Kiambu area the same term is used for a popular mash of githeri with potatoes, bananas and greens. Fruits are known as *matunda*, green leaves as *nyeni*. *Mboga* means cabbage but also denotes vegetables in general, including green leaves. Meat is called *nyama*; different kinds of meat are identified by reference to the particular animal. Similarly, *mutu* is flour and individual flours are named after the grains. Finally, *hindi* stands for all kinds of seeds and grains. There are no words for food groups such as legumes, roots and tubers, cereals or spices. The Kikuyu names of individual foods are given in Table 7 (Benson, 1964; Benson & Barlow, 1975; Blankhart, 1974b; NIRP, 1977).

A study of Kikuyu food classification nevertheless showed that six major food groups are distinguished: cereals, roots & tubers, legumes, vegetables, fruits, meats & animal products (HN, 1978a). Women seem to make no further divisions within these groups and there is also no indication that some groups are less clearly identified than others (Box F). Onions, peppers, carrots and tomatoes are an exception in that they are not associated with vegetables and do not belong to any other food group either. There are indications that maize and green bananas, two important staple foods, occupy a somewhat marginal position in their respective groups.

***Box F*. Food classification**

In a short study of the Kikuyu classificatory system mothers were asked to name the foods they regarded most similar to a series of 64 foods from 6 food groups that were read out one by one by the interviewer. Table F below lists the percentage of foods from the same or other food groups that were mentioned in response. On average, more than 76% of the replies consisted of foods from the same food group, indicating that the Kikuyu food classification does not differ from the nutritional assignation generally used.

Table F. *Foods regarded similar to each other (%)*

	Foods presented[1]					
	(1)	(2)	(3)	(4)	(5)	(6)
Responses[1]						
1. Cereals	**76**	6	3	3	–	1
2. Roots & tubers	8	**71**	2	5	5	2
3. Legumes	6	3	**78**	4	–	3
4. Vegetables	1	3	4	**76**	1	3
5. Fruits	–	6	–	–	**74**	–
6. Animal products	2	1	3	4	1	**81**
Miscellaneous	1	3	1	1	6	2
No response	6	7	9	7	13	8
Total	100	100	100	100	100	100

[1] Arranged by food group
Source: HN, 1980c

In general, Kikuyu mothers are reasonably familiar with important principles of child nutrition. They are able to recognize malnutrition and are aware of its nutritional causes although the nutritional nature of marasmus appears less well known than that of kwashiorkor. Most mothers prefer to breastfeed until the child reaches the age of about one year. Mothers generally consider it necessary to introduce various 'solid', 'supplementary' or 'weaning' foods quite early. Certain foods, such as gitoero, are introduced first, others later, such as ucuru and beans, while ngima with vegetables, for example, is not given until the end of the first year.

One of the causes underlying child malnutrition in Africa is the bulky nature of certain popular dishes, which makes it difficult to give children enough food during meal sittings (Church, 1979). Most Kikuyu mothers, however, are not aware of the need of multiple feedings, i.e. to let children eat frequently, and less than half the mothers in the NIRP-survey reported that (two-year-old) children were given anything in addition to the three main meals of the day. Present-day Kikuyu beliefs regarding diarrhoea are more in line with modern medical thinking. There is a general agreement that children should not be given milk in the case of diarrhoea but water with sugar and/or salt or plain water (HNS, 1984: 77).

In general, Kikuyu women have a high preference for legumes and animal products as foods for young children. Next follow vegetables, and roots & tubers, as shown by responses of mothers on a paired comparison schedule (a description of this schedule is given in Chapter 6.3). Figure 2 pictures the average percentage of mothers choosing animal products, legumes, vegetables, roots & tubers, and cereals on the occasions that these foods were presented. The low preference for cereals does not seem to accord with the large quantities of maize eaten by young children of all age groups. This may be because maize is regarded as the common staple.

Within the respective food groups there is again a certain order of preference. Among the cereals there is a high preference for millet flour which was traditionally used to prepare ucuru, a light porridge for children (although present-day consumption is low). Among meat and animal products preferences are related to tenderness; beef which is generally eaten rather tough is least preferred for children. Green bananas and Irish potatoes are more popular than sweet potatoes. Beans are the most popular legume;

Figure 2. *Maternal food preferences by food group (N=300)*

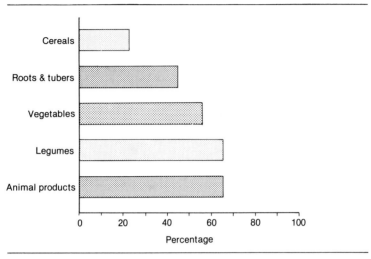

Source: HNS, 1984:37

kale and cabbage are most liked among the vegetables (HN, 1980c).

In general, women who have attended secondary school for some time are slightly more knowledgeable about child nutrition. They also have a higher preference for legumes and animal products, and express a lower preference for roots & tubers. Educated mothers, moreover, tend to stop breastfeeding at an earlier age, but they are also inclined to wait longer before introducing the child to the full adult diet, which means that children are fed on 'supplementary' or 'weaning' foods for a longer time (HNS, 1984: 38).

4.3 Child Food Consumption

The pattern of child feeding that has been described for many sedentary African populations is also found among the Kikuyu. Children usually receive the first supplementary food around the age of three months (CBS, 1983b). Different surveys place

Figure 3. *Daily food consumption of pre-school children (N=300; aged 6–59 months)*

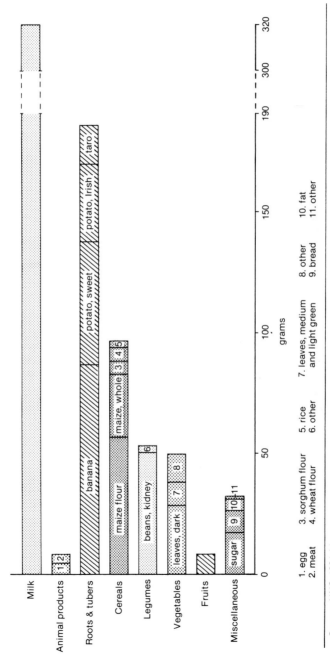

1. egg
2. meat

3. sorghum flour
4. wheat flour

5. rice
6. other

7. leaves, medium
   and light green

8. other
9. bread

10. fat
11. other

Source: HNS, 1984:44

the average duration of breastfeeding at 12–16 months, and the percentage of women that stop breastfeeding at an early age, before six months, is considered to be less than 25% (CBS, 1977; 1979; 1983b). From an early age, Kikuyu children are given large quantities of milk and tea to drink. National surveys have consistently shown that the frequency of milk consumption in Central Province is much higher than elsewhere in Kenya (CBS, 1981a).[3] Gitoero, bananas and potatoes mashed together and often prepared with milk to soften the texture is the favourite solid dish for young children. Its importance decreases as children grow older. At young ages ngima (stiff maize porridge) and ucuru (light porridge) are next in importance. The consumption of ngima increases as children grow older but the consumption of ucuru remains more or less constant during the first years of life. Young children are not given githeri, the dish of maize and beans, because it is prepared with whole maize kernels which are regarded as unsuitable for young children. Mothers introduce this dish by serving the children the beans and no, or only some token, maize. Only later, from the age of two onwards, are they given proportionally more maize. Gradually during the third and fourth year a shift occurs towards the adult diet. By the age of four most children not only eat with the adults but also eat the same meals, although they may still be given some extras, such as ucuru when prepared for younger siblings.

The NIRP-survey collected detailed data on the consumption of dishes, foods, food groups and the energy and protein intake of pre-school children, particularly concentrating on children aged two years.[4] Among pre-school children, the quantity of milk consumed is by far the largest of any single ingredient.[5] This is followed by roots & tubers, cereals, legumes and vegetables (Figure 3; detailed data are listed in Appendix 1, which also presents figures on the frequency of consumption). Among the group of roots & tubers, green banana is eaten most, followed by sweet potato and Irish potato. Maize flour and whole maize account for most of the cereal consumption. The traditional grains, sorghum and millet, are less important for child diets.[6] Kidney beans account for nearly all of the legumes; dark leaves (kale) for most of the vegetable consumption. The amounts of animal products and fruits eaten are small, and daily only four grams of fat are used on average.

Figure 4. *Daily consumption of food groups by pre-school children*

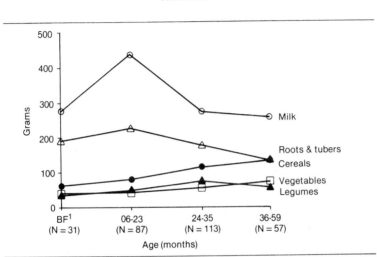

[1] BF = Children, aged 6-23 months, breastfeeding, breastmilk consumption not included.
Source: HNS, 1984:45

Breakdown of the NIRP-survey results by age group shows that milk consumption is highest among young children who are no longer breastfed (Figure 4).[7] Young children eat relatively large amounts of roots & tubers but later on this decreases substantially, while the consumption of foods from other food groups increases. Legume consumption peaks among the two-year olds, and cereals account for an increasing share of the daily intake with age.

Energy and protein intake reaches a fairly high level among the one-year-olds but, surprisingly, remains more or less constant among the older age groups (Figure 5). Although milk and roots & tubers compose the bulk of the raw foodstuffs, the smaller amounts of cereals that are consumed contribute most to energy intake: 31% on average for all age groups combined. It is followed in importance by roots & tubers (19%) and milk (19%), while legumes constitute the fourth source of energy (16%). Protein intake is, first of all, provided by legumes (33%), next by milk (28%), and in this respect cereals take third position, with 23% of the total.

Figure 5. *Source of energy and protein intake by food group*

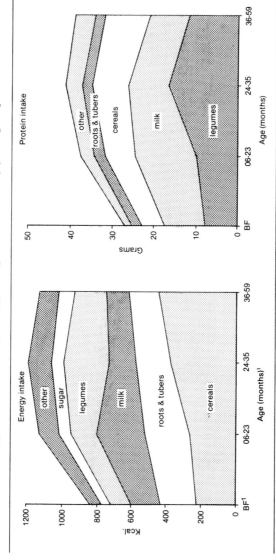

[1]Information on age group composition is listed with Figure 4.
Source: HNS, 1984:47

Figure 6. *Daily energy and protein intake of pre-school children per kg body weight*

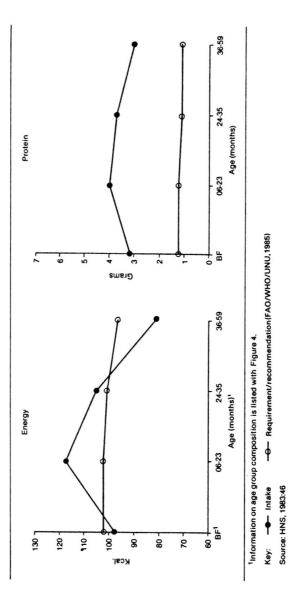

Key: —●— Intake   —○— Requirement/recommendation(FAO/WHO/UNU,1985)

Source: HNS, 1983:46

[1] Information on age group composition is listed with Figure 4.

Figure 6 presents the intakes in relative terms, i.e. per kilogram body weight and compared with international recommendations (WHO, 1985). Breastmilk consumption was not measured but the supplementary foods already cover recommended protein and as much as 90% of energy requirements among the breastfed children. (Although these figures may well be lower among the youngest children in this group, below twelve months of age.) Among the one-year-olds energy and protein intake surpasses the WHO recommendations for children of this age, even though these norms themselves are often considered to be rather high. Energy intake, however, decreases relatively with age and, in fact, for elder children falls below the required daily intake. Protein intake shows the same trend but remains above recommendations. These data correspond with similar findings reported for Akamba children (Steenbergen, Kusin & Jansen, 1984) and Luo children (Niemeyer et al., 1985). In both studies the same trends of satisfactory protein intakes and a relative decrease in energy intakes were noted.

Differences in food consumption exist between children from different households. There is strong evidence of a relation between energy intake and income group, but no systematic differences seem to exist between households from different areas, at different domestic stages, or with different numbers of young children. Protein intake does not show any significant variations corresponding with any of these environmental factors, and remains uniformly high.

Differences in energy intake appear to occur mainly among the one- and two-year-olds, with children from rich households having a considerably higher intake than children from other households (Figure 7). At the particularly vulnerable age of one year, children from rich households consumed 1350kcal, children from medium households 1150kcal and from poor households only 900kcal. The lower energy intake is due to a lesser intake of cereals and milk at that age, and although there is a tendency among poor households to compensate for this by giving more legumes, this compensation occurs mainly among the two-year-olds, and not yet at the age of one year. Thus differences in nutrition between income groups are not simply a matter of more or less, but of differences in nutritional patterns that are often complementary in nature.

No differences in energy intake were found between the two survey locations. There are, however, some differences in the

Figure 7. *Daily energy intake of pre-school children by income group*

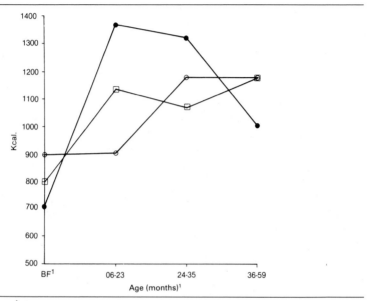

[1]Information on age group composition is listed with Figure 4.

Key (households): ●—rich   ☐—medium   ⊖—poor

Source: HNS, 1984: 54

composition of the diet that conform with the known differences in agriculture. In the lower location milk consumption is less and the consumption of roots & tubers is higher, although it should be noted that these differences were smallest among the youngest age groups, which underscores the importance of these foods as weaning foods.

Neither were differences in energy and protein intake found to exist between families at different domestic stages or families differing in number of pre-school children. And, although formal education has a positive influence on nutritional cognition, the educational level of the mother was not related to actual food consumption. Apparently child diets are not so much decided by family composition or individual cognition of the mother as by prevailing cultural patterns and the availability of resources.

4.4 Nutritional State of Young Children

Since 1960, several surveys of the nutritional state of young children have been held in Central Province, but results are not easy to compare because of differences in location and time (Table 8). There is also considerable variation in the age range and the number of children surveyed. The manner and quality of reporting also vary, although most surveys relate their findings to the Harvard reference standards using the indicators weight-for-age (W-A), height-for-age (H-A) and weight-for-height (W-H). It is generally agreed that W-H indicates the momentary nutritional condition of children, that H-A mainly reflects previous nutritional history, while W-A serves as general, combined index of nutritional status.

Rodriguez (1972) reported that more than 60% of children were below W-H (90) and below W-A (80). This survey was held in a location in Murang'a District. An earlier survey in 1965 found that 40% of children were below W-H (90) in five locations in Murang'a and Nyeri District (Bohdall et al., n.d.). These studies, however, cover only small numbers of children and the first studies with larger samples reported more favourable findings (Korte, 1969; Korte & Simmons, 1972). Later surveys also reported fewer children falling below critical values of H-A and W-H. The NIRP-survey reported a mean height-for-age of 93, and a mean weight-for-height of 96, with 20% of the children falling below H-A (90) and a similar percentage below W-H (90) (the major anthropometric results of the NIRP-survey are listed in Appendices 2 and 3). The most recent CBS survey of 1982 reported an average height-for-age of 94.6 and an average weight-for-height of 99.1. In most surveys since 1975 the percentage of stunted children (below H-A (90)) tends to be between 20 and 25% and the percentage of wasted children (below W-H (90)) around 20%.

Systematic comparison of data from the three CBS surveys between 1976 and 1982 gave no consistent evidence of changes in

Table 8. *Review of child nutrition surveys in Central Province*

Survey reference	Year of survey	District	Number of children	Age range (months)	Weight-for-age		Height-for-age		Weight-for-height		
					average (s.d.)	% below W-A(80)	average (s.d.)	% below H-A(90)	average (s.d.)	% below W-H(90)	% below W-H(80)
Bohdal, Gibbs & Simmons (n.d.)	1965	Murang'a; Nyeri	90[1]	0–59	—	—	—	—	—	40	9.0
Korte (1969)	1966	Kirinyaga	308/371	1–96	82	—	92	—	95	—	—
Korte & Simmons (1972)	1969	Nyeri	130	6–74	85	—	94	—	96	—	—
Rodrigues (1972)	1971	Murang'a	64	0–59	—	61	—	—	—	64	33.9
O'Keefe (1978)	1974	Murang'a	125	0–36	—	27	—	—	—	—	—
CBS (1977)	1977	All districts	225	12–48	84	39	93	31	94	33	3.0
Hoorweg, Niemeyer & Steenbergen (1983)[2]	1978	Murang'a	508	6–59	86 (10.3)	28	93 (4.5)	21	96 (7.8)	22	1.5
CBS (1979a)	1978/9	All districts	300	6–60	—	23	—	22	—	20	2.4
CBS (1983b)	1982	All districts	907	3–60	—	—	94.6 (6.5)	20	99.1 (10.9)	17	2.8

[1] Estimated figure. The children in 62 families were examined; exact number of children not reported.
[2] NIRP-survey

nutritional status during that period (CBS, 1983b: 25). Never-theless, the general impression is that over the last twenty years improvements have been achieved. On the other hand, it must be mentioned that although children from elite schools in Nairobi show virtually the same height results as a reference population (CBS, 1979a), rural Kikuyu children clearly remain below this level. Apparently the growth of Kikuyu children is less than optimal, although the loss does not assume extreme proportions.

The national figures show that the nutritional status of children in Central Province does not differ substantially from that of children elsewhere in Kenya. Although the first national survey indicated that the percentage of stunted children in Central Province was second highest, after Eastern Province, some doubts have since been expressed about these findings. The more recent surveys of 1978 and 1982, with larger samples of children, indicate that the provinces with the greater number of nutritional problem cases are Coast and Nyanza Province, and that children in Central Province are near the national average or even slightly above (Table 9).

Table 9. *Results of national surveys of child nutrition by province*

	Average H-A		Percentage below H-A(90)	
	1979	1982	1979	1982
Central	94.5	94.0	21	24
Coast	92.9	92.2	40	39
Eastern	94.6	93.3	24	27
Nyanza	93.6	93.4	34	33
Rift Valley	94.2	94.9	24	22
Western	94.0	92.9	24	30
National	94.5	93.7	27	28

Source: CBS, 1983b

4.5 Ecological and Household Variations

It is usually assumed that differences in ecology are an important contributory factor in the condition of children, and that the nutritional status of children is lower in areas with less ecological potential. Data cited in support of this assumption are usually drawn from Mbithi & Wisner (1972) and CBS (1979b). The first study showed a steady increase in children with low weights (less than W-A (70)) in zones at different altitudes in Eastern Province; 10% in the highest zone and 35% in the very lowest zone. However, this survey, which was restricted to children of three years and younger, did not take height measures, and the results may also reflect temporary conditions resulting from the years of drought preceding the time of the survey. The CBS report (1979b) contains an analysis of height-for-age, a more reliable indicator of long-term nutritional conditions, and compares results for ecological zones, on the basis of data from the First National Nutrition Survey in 1976. Although the general conclusion was that the proportion of nutritionally small children increases steadily in lower zones from 20% to 40%, there are inconsistencies in the findings that indicate that this trend is, at least, not general for all of Kenya.

Restricting the analysis to the general region in which Central Province is situated, east of Rift Valley, the average H-A of children by ecological zone is as listed in Table 10. If anything,

Table 10. *Central Province: Nutritional status by ecological zone (average H-A)*

	Ecological zone				
	2 (tea)	2/3	3 (coffee)	3/4	4 (cotton)
CBS, 1979b[1]	93.0	—	92.0	—	95.7
HN, 1980a[2]	94.7	—	95.7	—	94.7
HNS, 1983[2]	—	93.1	—	93.1	—

[1] Children: aged 12–48 months
[2] Children: aged 6–59 months

the children in the lower area have the most satisfactory condition.[8] The two other studies listed in Table 10 are limited to locations in Central Province. The results firstly concern pre-school children visiting the health centres in the three study areas, situated at considerable distances from each other.[9] Many of these children attended in connection with health complaints; this could have affected weight-for-height but not height-for-age, and the results therefore do not indicate systematic differences in nutritional condition (HN, 1980a). The most systematic comparison, however, is provided by the NIRP-survey, conducted in two different ecological zones, in survey locations about 25km from each other on the mountain slopes. No difference in average H-A was observed between children aged 6–59 months in the two areas (HNS, 1983).

One explanation of this discrepancy between national and provincial trends is that in Central Province, ecological zone and farm size are related, as described in Chapter 3. Households compensate for less favourable agricultural conditions by increasing their farm size and by off-farm employment as described earlier. In these circumstances differences in nutritional conditions can no longer be expected from crude comparison between areas. A similar finding was, in fact, reported from Machakos District; anthropometric examinations of Akamba children in two nearby but different ecological areas did not reveal differences in nutritional status either (Oomen et al., 1979). The ecological differences covered in the NIRP-survey (and the Akamba study) were relatively small and certainly did not represent ecological extremes. Nevertheless, the comparison still covers the range of ecological conditions under which most of the population in Central Province lives. This suggests that in Central Province there exists by and large a balance at least as far as the nutritional state of young children is concerned between, on the one hand, the needs of the population and, on the other, income from agricultural production and off-farm employment. It would seem, therefore, that the differences in nutritional status of children probably have more to do with differences between households than between ecological conditions.

The CBS report (1979b) further analyzed the relation between household conditions and nutritional state of young children by means of a regression analysis and presents a profile of sub-groups with statistically higher rates of protein–energy malnutrition (low H-A), as follows:

> The household operates a holding (cultivates land); dry season water source is neither a lake nor a still pool, but is less than 2km. from the holding; the head of household is male; he is not employed in health/education/welfare, as an agricultural labourer, or in an urban

occupation; the holding area is less than 5 hectares, 1 to 3 hectares were initially planted and no cattle are on the holding (CBS, 1979b: 2).

In the subgroup with all these characteristics, nearly 50% of the children were stunted and were below H-A (90). It is worth noticing that the chances of childhood malnutrition increase where the head of the household has no employment and farm size is small. The analysis, however, suffered from the disadvantage that no differentiation was made between different population groups, so that cultural differences must have caused considerable variation in conditions and nutritional practices.[10] Subsequent analysis of the same data indicated that in Central Province there are differences in the prevalence of stunting between children of small and children of large farmers (Haaga et al., 1985).

The NIRP-survey used a different frame of analysis, first identifying the major factors on which Kikuyu households differ and subsequently relating these to the nutritional status of children. The major determining factors are income group, domestic stage and number of young children, and findings regarding the relation with nutritional status are given in Figure 8. Income group is clearly the most important factor: the greatest differences in height-for-age occur between children from poor and rich households. The greater resources of rich households clearly benefit the young children. As we saw in the previous section, energy intake similarly varies with household resources. The relation between income group and nutritional status thus appears to be fairly straight-forward (Box G).

The role of family composition is less clearcut and less easy to understand. There are differences in nutritional status correspond-ing with domestic stage and number of young children, but these differences are small and there are no antecedent relations with food consumption. Indications are that peer pressure among young children has a negative effect and that an explanation for this must probably be sought in the quality of child care. Young children place the greatest burden on the mother and in households with many young children mothers can give less individual attention to each child, or not enough when it is most needed as in the case of illness. Other explanations, however, cannot be ruled out, notably that the presence of several young children may increase the risk of infection. The findings in respect of domestic stage also indicate

Figure 8. *Average height-for-age of pre-school children by income group, domestic stage & number of pre-school children in household*

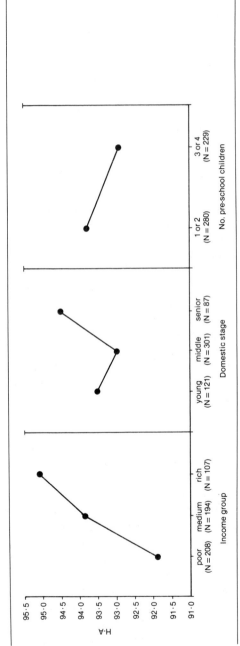

Source: HNS, 1983:63

70

Box G. **Commercialization of agriculture**

There is a widespread opinion that the cultivation of cashcrops detracts from foodcrop cultivation and that this is one of the main causes underlying malnutrition. The relation between export crop production and the nutritional status of the population, however, is much more complicated and depends on mediating factors such as ecological potential, agricultural cycles, availability of land, labour and agricultural inputs, prices and income distribution (Fleuret & Fleuret, 1980; Tosh, 1980; Pinstrup-Andersen, 1983).

The NIRP-survey found that in the rural areas of Central Province there was a positive relation between income group (defined on the basis of degree of commercial farming and off-farm employment) and nutritional status. An analysis of national survey data for the whole of Kenya did not find evidence that cash-crop cultivation influences the nutritional state of young children negatively (CBS, 1979b; Haaga et al., 1985). In a way this is quite understandable. Children from well-to-do households are generally in better condition, and these are also the households with more resources, and therefore more involved in cash-crop cultivation. Alternatively, it is sometimes suggested that cash-crop cultivation is particularly damaging in the case of poor households with few resources, who are tempted to use all or most of their land for commercial cultivation, leaving not enough land for subsistence purposes.

Data on the households of women admitted with malnourished children at FLT centres, however, do not confirm this suggestion. Taking into account differences in farm size it turned out that the extent of coffee cultivation among these households was less than that of households in the control group.

Table G. *Households cultivating cash crops (%)*

| | *Farm size (acres)* | | | |
	no land	0.1–0.9	1.0–2.9	3.0 or more
FLT-cases	–	0	30	41
Control group	–	30	48	79

Source: HN, 1982: 81

that the age composition of children plays a crucial role. Children from senior families are in better condition, and more detailed analysis has shown that this is related to the presence of grown-up children (HNS, 1983: 64). Children over seventeen years are expected to contribute their labour to the household, thus providing an additional resource, but they can also give direct help with various household chores and the care of young children.

How strongly the three above mentioned factors work out in combination, i.e. the interactions between income group, domestic stage and number of young children, is best demonstrated by the incidence of children at risk, in this case children with low weights (Figure 9). Among the NIRP-survey population as a whole, 28% of the children were below W-A (80) but this percentage fluctuates strongly depending on the actual combination of conditions. A first, general inspection of the curves shows that the effect of income group is consistent under nearly all conditions; similarly the effect when families have to raise several children of pre-school age. It is also evident that senior families form a more favourable environment than young families, but that the results for middle-stage families are not consistent. The incidence of children at risk, however, rises dramatically for certain combinations of conditions, notably when poor households have to care for several pre-school children, an interaction that is independent of domestic stage and which results in more than 60% of the young children being below W-A (80). At the other end of the spectrum, in rich households consisting of senior families with few pre-school children, none of the children was found at risk. The most unfavourable combination of conditions is encountered in poor households consisting of young families with three or more children of pre-school age, a group in which over 80% of the children were found to be of low weight. These figures provide a striking demonstration of the importance of the respective economic and social factors for the nutritional status of children. There are also indications that the children in poor households experience strong weight variations of a seasonal nature. Weight records at Pre-School Health clinics over a three-year period revealed that W-A dropped from an average of 90% for the period December–February to an average of 80% in the period August–October (Hitchings, 1979). These variations can make children the more susceptible to episodes of acute malnutrition.

Figure 9. *Percentage of pre-school children below W-A(80) by income group × domestic stage × number of pre-school children in household*

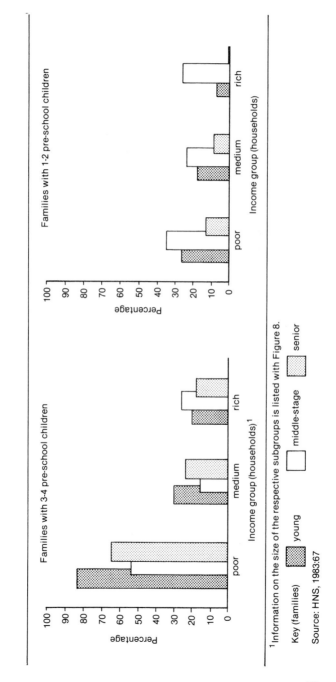

4.6 Aetiology of Childhood Malnutrition

The social and economic factors that influence nutritional status may, alone or in combination, contribute to more severe forms of childhood malnutrition, as the incidence of children with low weights in certain households indicates. Nevertheless, not all severe cases of malnutrition are necessarily characterized by the same combination of conditions. Children may be the victim of individual circumstances, or they may belong to special, disadvantaged groups. General surveys usually do not give sufficient information on this, particularly when the incidence of malnutrition is low and the number of cases in the community at a specific point in time small. Study of malnourished cases may throw additional light on this; and in the present case the Family Life Training Centres offer that opportunity.

Comparison of women admitted to FLT-centres in Central Province with a control group selected from the general population (for description, see p. 94), shows that the groups differ in a number of social and economic characteristics (Table 11). The first group are predominantly from poor households, many have no farm land, they are less educated, many women are unmarried,

Table 11. *Protein–energy malnutrition: Case characteristics*

	FLT Cases[1] (N=85)	Control group (N=100)
Income group (% poor households)	67	42
Domestic stage (% young families)	26	24
Pre-school children (% with 3 or more p-s children)	43	35
Education, mother (% without formal education)	59	34
Marital status, mother (% unmarried)	27	8
Farm size (% without land)	36	0

[1] Cases admitted to Family Life Training Centres
Source: HN, 1982: 82

either single but more often separated, and they have more pre-school children. The characteristics of poverty and peer pressure are in line with the previous findings, and so is the lesser education because this is a common characteristic of low income groups. However, the additional differences indicate that marital instability and landlessness are also important factors, at least in Central Province. These groups are often under-represented in general surveys because they tend to stay together in population pockets, for instance on or near large agricultural estates or shopping centres, rather than living evenly spread out among the total population.

On the whole, the women admitted with malnourished children are less educated, but they are not less knowledgeable about child nutrition. If anything, they appeared to be slightly better informed and also showed a general preference for high-energy/high-protein foods (see Table 17, p. 106). As will be argued later, these women have probably become sensitized in the course of the illness of the child. Whatever the reason for this raised level of awareness, there are no indications that lack of nutritional knowledge or poor maternal preferences are an important cause of malnutrition among this group, at least in this part of Kenya (Box H).

About 30% of the women are not or no longer married, which is almost three times the incidence among the rural population. In the previous chapter it was already pointed out that divorced women often find themselves in a very difficult position. Sometimes these women can move in with their parents, or live at the sufferance of one of their brothers. Others have to find employment, which is not easy in the rural areas; they may find work as permanent labourers at agricultural estates but more often they have to exist on earnings from casual labour. Others work as barmaids and some turn to prostitution; there are even cases of rural homeless and destitutes.

But not only unmarried women are among the destitute, there are also other rural poor, notably the landless families. About half the FLT-cases have no land or less than an acre at their disposal and often they have no land to grow food crops. Very few of the women at FLT centres (about 25%) reported that they were able to grow enough food to feed their families, and even fewer that they had milk or eggs available from home production. They also have few opportunities for commercial farming and often these women lack the income from regular employment of a husband.

***Box H*. Aetiology of childhood malnutrition**

The case studies in this monograph are drawn from Central Province. There are strong indications that the aetiology of malnutrition in Western Kenya is somewhat different. In Central Province relatively many of the women with malnourished children admitted to the FLT centres are not or no longer married, have no land at their disposal and have to engage in casual labour for their livelihood. Comparison with the cases admitted at FLT centres in Western Kenya reveals that a higher proportion of women there are young, have only one child to look after and are pregnant.

It appears therefore that in Western Kenya the causation of childhood malnutrition tends to be linked with factors such as inexperience of mothers, traditional feeding practices and child rearing practices. The family structure in Western Kenya, furthermore, differs from that in Central Province in the sense that families are more often extended in type with more sharing of responsibility for children. There is also a higher incidence of polygamy, a factor which is often pointed at as another major contributing factor to childhood malnutrition.

It is true that in Western Kenya more children were brought to the FLT centres by persons other than their mother, while more of the mothers were polygamously married. It is also true that the rate of polygamy is higher than among the general population in this part of Kenya so that it indeed appears a minor contributing factor. A suggested explanation for this is the fact that young women who marry in polygamous unions are traditionally given heavy workloads and are expected to assist their elder co-wives and/or mothers-in-law.

The above remarks are concerned with the causation of severe malnutrition, but they should not be taken to suggest that in this part of Kenya no relationship exists between household income and nutritional status of children. A recent study among rice cultivators in Western Kenya found that the nutritional status of children improves with greater diversification of household resources (Niemeijer et al., 1985; 1988). However, this study also found that there were relatively few cases of acute malnutrition among the lowest income group, which suggests that additional triggering mechanisms have to be taken into account.

Box H cont.

Table H. *Characteristics of mothers at FLT centres, 1978 (%)*

	Central Province[1]	*Western Kenya*[2]
Age, 29 years or younger	47	68
Looking after 1 child only	10	17
Pregnant	17	28
Single, separated, divorced or widowed	38	12
Married in polygamous union	16	41
No farmland	43	7
Engaged in casual labour	59	6

[1] Kiambu, Murang'a, Kirinyaga FLTC
[2] Bungoma, Busia, Kisumu FLTC
Source: HN, 1979

Under these circumstances, they are often under the same pressure as unmarried women to earn an income through casual labour.

In summary, major background factors in the causation of childhood malnutrition appear to be marital instability, land-lessness and concurrent lack of resources. These factors tend to occur in combination although the bottleneck in most cases is poverty, which, apart from a lack of resources, means extra work for women who often lack an economic provider and, at the same time, a protector of their economic interests. Problems of poverty and heavy workloads are at the very root of childhood malnutrition in this part of Kenya.

Chapter 5

Nutrition Intervention in Central Province

Already from an early date the nutritional conditions in Central Province were a matter of concern. The Kikuyu served as suppliers of grain to the exploratory expeditions and early traders in East Africa (Rogers, 1979), but there is also repeated mention of famines (Cranworth, 1939) and of malnutrition among destitute individuals and households (Paterson, 1943). An important responsibility of the colonial administration, early in the century, was to secure the food supply of the region, to regulate the food trade, and to set up relief programmes in cases of emergency. Initially relief programmes tended to be incidental in times of famines, but later they became institutionalized. Since 1950, when attention of health workers started to focus on childhood malnutrition, nutrition intervention was increasingly aimed at young children. It was developed along three different lines: first of all, the treatment and care of cases of protein–energy malnutrition; secondly, food aid to children from poor and destitute families (particularly during the social upheaval of the Emergency in the 1950s); and thirdly, general prevention in the form of nutrition education as part of the general health services. The major existing nutrition programmes clearly reflect these three developments. The Nutrition Field Workers represent the general

Table 12. *Characteristics of child nutrition programmes and NIRP study areas*

Programme	Target group, type intervention & exposure	Study area	Programme site	Description	Attendance during 1978	Reports
Nutrition Field Workers	all pre-school children; nutrition education; irregular visits;	Limuru	Lari	Health Centre with visiting NFW	not available	Campbell, 1975 HN, 1980a
		Kandara	Kandara	Health Centre with permanent NFW	not available	
		Mwea	Kimbimbi	Health Centre with permanent NFW	not available	
Pre-school Health Programme	needy households; food supplementation & nutrition education; 1 visit per month;	Limuru	Kereita	Mission Maternity	250 children	CRS, 1972 HN, 1980b
		Kandara	Gaichanjiru	Mission Hospital	500 children	
		Mwea	Karaba	Mission without medical facilities	500 children	
Family Life Training Centres	malnourished children; nutrition rehabilitation; 3-week course;	Limuru	Limuru	8 cottages	73 mothers + 227 children	Gachuhi et al. 1972 MoHSS, 1976–79 HN, 1977, 1979, 1982 Niemeyer, 1982 AMREF, 1978, 1979, 1980 Poskitt, 1979
		Kandara	Kigumo	16 cottages	126 mothers + 288 children	
		Mwea	Wamugu	8 rooms	74 mothers + 159 children	

educational approach, the Pre-School Health Programme is a food supplementation programme and the Family Life Training Centres belong to the category of nutrition rehabilitation centres. Further description of the programmes and of our study locations follows below; the major characteristics of the programmes and the selected clinics are summarized in Table 12.

5.1 Nutrition Field Workers

Nutrition Field Workers are registered nurses who have followed a six-month nutrition course at Karen College, Nairobi. In 1978 there were about 160 stationed throughout the country, evenly distributed over the seven provinces, with the exception of North-Eastern province where only five Field Workers were active. Roughly two-thirds of the Field Workers are stationed at hospitals and about one-third at health centres. They are responsible to the District Medical Officers and the Provincial Nutritionists, who receive monthly reports of their activities. The number of families reached by the average Field Worker per year was estimated at 2500 (Campbell, 1975). The effectiveness of the programme reportedly suffered from administrative difficulties concerning deployment of personnel, organizational support, supervision and lack of transport.

The principal task of the Nutrition Field Workers is to contribute to the regular maternal and child health (MCH) services. They are expected to see the children that are brought to the clinic, to check their weights and nutritional status in general, to identify malnourished children for special attention, to give nutritional advice to mothers and, finally, to give some nutrition instruction to the group of mothers at large, mostly in the form of a lecture-cum-demonstration. This kind of work is not restricted to the hospital or health centre where they are stationed: on certain days of the week they may function as members of the MCH team at a health centre where no Nutrition Field Worker is stationed permanently, or as members of a mobile MCH team. A second task of the Field Workers is to pay regular visits to homes in the area in order to follow the progress of previous cases of malnutrition, other borderline cases and children at risk. A third duty is to keep an eye on the kitchen of the hospital or health centre, if present, and check on cleanliness, menus and special diets.

In practice, the Nutrition Field Workers have individual freedom to organize their activities and as a result their work shows considerable variation. The activities of the Field Workers and other MCH personnel overlap and some Field Workers perform mainly MCH activities such as immunization, and have little time left for their nutritional duties. Others, however, insist on their specific role, sometimes isolating themselves from other members of the MCH team who have different expectations of them. The lecture-cum-demonstration, generally considered the core of the fieldworkers' activities, is in many cases given irregularly and infrequently. Some Field Workers make a serious effort at home-visiting but the actual coverage and effectiveness of these visits are often disappointing (HN, 1980a).

Patient administration at health centres is minimal: no records were kept of individual mothers or children. The Field Workers therefore had little systematic information about the attendance patterns and social characteristics of visitors to the health centre, and they had to rely on their individual experience and the insights they had gained locally. Unfortunately, the turnover rate among the Field Workers is high; many of them are young women, about to get married or already married and they tend to follow their (future) husbands.

The rural health centres at Lari, Kandara and Kimbimbi were selected for the evaluation studies. At the two latter centres Nutrition Field Workers had been stationed for more than five years. In Lari the field worker of the nearby Limuru health centre had been participating in the weekly MCH clinic for several years. The MCH services in Kandara had long been integrated; in Lari this had happened more recently, while in Kimbimbi there was no integration of services yet.

5.2 Pre-School Health Programme

Catholic Relief Services (CRS) sponsors child nutrition pro-grammes in a number of developing countries. The objective of the Pre-School Health (PSH) programme is to maintain adequate growth of the pre-school children in the communities concerned by educating mothers in child care, by periodic assessment of the children's nutritional progress, and by providing supplementary foods (CRS–USCC; PCI, 1980). In Kenya, this means that Catholic Relief Services imports foods received through USAID. This food is delivered free of charge at the port of arrival, Mombasa. CRS–Kenya distributes the food to the participating agencies, half of them Catholic mission hospitals, the rest government health facilities, other missions and some private organizations. These institutions are obliged to organize special clinics (here called PSH clinics) for mothers and children. These clinics are limited in size, not more than 60 children per session is the rule, and each session takes a full morning or afternoon. Clinics can hold between four and twenty sessions a month.[1] The clinics are run by two, three or four assistants, depending on local circumstances. The assistants usually consist of locally recruited personnel with a few years of secondary education and who have been given on-the-spot training. In 1979 there were some 135 PSH clinics in Kenya, with about 45,000 children enrolled.

Enrolment in PSH clinics is possible for children between six months and five years (60 months) of age. In Kenya the programme policy is to give priority to children from poor, needy families. The actual selection of mothers and children is left to the participating agency. Mother and child are required to attend once a month on a fixed day. If they do not attend for three consecutive months, without good reason, they are dropped from the programme. Once a child reaches the age of five it can no longer participate in the programme but its place is often taken by a younger sibling from the same family, so that a family can participate much longer than a particular child. New mothers seeking entrance to the programme often have to remain on the waiting list for a long time before a place becomes available. Sometimes mothers, in really desperate circumstances, may try to force admission to the programme by repeatedly attending all morning, even though not receiving any foods. If she persists, she is eventually given a place. There comes a point, however, when all places have been given out and the only alternative remaining to the clinic staff is to organize one more session a month.

The clinics are usually held during the morning and the average mother spends about two hours at the clinic, three quarters of this time being spent waiting.[2] Upon arrival the child is weighed and the weight is recorded in the clinic records as well as on the weight chart which is kept by the mother. The mother may also be given some individual advice while the child's weight is recorded. Next, she joins the other mothers to wait until all are present, after which a lecture-cum-demonstration is given. The teaching assistants usually have a fixed repertory of lectures on child care. Child nutrition is given relatively much attention, particularly the preparation of the foods that are distributed at the clinics. After the lecture the food rations are distributed, which usually consists of several pounds of corn–soya mixture or dried skimmed milk, bulgar wheat and oil.[3] For this, a mother contributes about five shillings per child per month to cover local overhead costs and transport costs within Kenya. Since a few years, mothers have been allowed to enrol more than one child and may even become recipients of the programme themselves.[4] In that case, however, they are also charged double or three times the fee, i.e. 10 or 15 shillings, and it is doubtful whether the really poor are able to afford this.

Staff from the national CRS headquarters pay regular field visits to check the way the clinics function. The weight charts of children, taken in when the children reach the age of five, are collected regularly by staff from CRS headquarters and are occasionally analyzed (CRS, 1972). By and large, the PSH clinics seem to function as expected. Children are weighed, lectures given, food distributed, and most mothers attend every month. Few mothers drop out and absence rates among the regular participants are low, except when no food is available for distribution (as was the case for several months in 1977, when the monthly clinics were kept going but attendance rates dropped sharply, only to pick up again after food had arrived). One reservation, however, must be made. Very little individual advice appears to be given, and the average time per individual case of less than two minutes during which the child is also weighed, speaks for itself.

In Central Province there were about 30 PSH clinics in 1978, each with between 200 and 1000 children, and one centre, near Nairobi, where 1800 children were enrolled. In all, more than 17,500 children were enrolled in the Central Province programme. Three PSH clinics, situated in rural areas, were selected for the present study: Kereita Catholic Mission Maternity, Gaichanjiru Catholic Mission Hospital and Karaba Catholic Mission.

Kereita Maternity, situated in Kambaa village, had an enrolment of about 250 children but had doubled its intake by the end of our studies. Gaichanjiru Hospital had an enrolment of about 500 children which remained more or less constant. The PSH clinic at Karaba mission had been operating with ups and downs for several years but at the start of our studies, in 1977, an assistant was employed full-time and enrolment did rise to more than 500. By the end of 1978, however, some months after our interviews had ended, this clinic was closed down because of personnel problems and differences of opinion between the Kenya headquarters and the local agency.

5.3 Family Life Training Centres

During 1974–75 the Department of Social Services took charge of several nutrition clinics in Central and Western Kenya, which until then had been managed by voluntary organizations. The clinics were slightly reorganized and renamed Family Life Training (FLT) Centres. The objectives of the FLT programmes are to provide assistance, mainly in the form of education, to families that have, in official terms, 'not been able to maintain a healthy and productive life for their members' (MoHSS, 1980). Mothers with severely malnourished children are admitted together possibly with siblings of the children who are usually also in poor condition. They are admitted for the duration of a three-week course, unless the condition of the child shows no improvement, in which case they can stay on for some more time. The emphasis at the centres is on the treatment of childhood malnutrition.

During the period 1976–79 the national programme went through a rapid development and the number of admissions more than doubled: to 1700 mothers and 3000 children. The recurrent expenditures for 1978 were estimated at 300KSh per child. The three centres in Western Kenya had most admissions, and took care of three times the number of cases in Central Province (HN, 1979).

Each centre is equipped to house a number of mothers with malnourished children. Mothers are encouraged also to bring their other (young) children because siblings are often in poor condition as well. The centres are staffed with a supervisor, an assistant supervisor, and one or two house mothers, the latter usually being untrained personnel. The women remain at the centres for about three weeks; if improvement is not satisfactory after that period, mother and child may stay longer. Accommodation is usually designed in a local style and built from locally available materials. The mothers are expected to do the usual household chores such as cooking and cleaning just as they would at home, and also to work in the vegetable gardens attached to most of the centres and to look after any small livestock. During the stay at the centre the emphasis is on verbal and practical instruction in nutrition, as well as other aspects of child care and family life, such as sanitation, home management and family planning.

The three FLT centres in Central Province are situated in Kiambu, Murang'a and Kirinyaga districts. The centres in the first two districts were founded by the Kenya Red Cross in the 1950s, as centres for aid to poor families, in connection with the upheaval at the time of the Emergency. Later they were turned into nutrition rehabilitation centres, until they were finally handed over to the Department of Social Services. They offer accommodation in the form of roundavel cottages, 8 and 16 of them respectively. Kirinyaga FLTC was founded in 1976 and, at the time, offered accommodation in wooden houses that comprised 8 rooms altogether. During 1978 the three centres together admitted 275 mothers and 675 children, which is less than 40% of capacity.[5] In all, 135 children were admitted below W-A (60), which is far below the estimated number of cases of malnutrition in the three districts, and even below the number in the three divisions in which the centres are located. Conservative estimates place the number of malnourished children at any time at 1500 in the three districts combined and at 300 malnourished children in the three divisions.[6] The reasons for this under-utilization are not quite evident, although it must be noted that the centres carry the stigma of poor relief and do not have a favourable reputation among the population in general. They are further located at considerable distances, some 20–40km away, from the district medical headquarters so that cases are not easily referred.

5.4 Catchment Population

Table 13 lists various characteristics of women and children frequenting the three programmes;[7] some of the information regarding the FLT-cases has already been discussed in the previous chapter. The geographical catchment area of the PSH programme is relatively small, no doubt because the participants are required to visit monthly. The catchment area of the MCH services is somewhat larger, although most visitors still come from within a 5km radius. Although FLT centres draw their clients from a larger area, most cases still come from within the division in which the centres are situated, rather than from the district as a whole.

Among the MCH-visitors there are relatively many single girls and young married women, who also tend to be slightly better educated than average. The PSH-participants differ little from the general population, except that there are relatively many women who have not received any formal education. Among the FLT-cases there are even more women without schooling, while about 25% of these cases are not or no longer married and presumably have to manage largely on their own.

As regards family characteristics, MCH-visitors relatively often belong to young or senior families; this is a result of the presence of many young married women and single mothers. Young married women have by definition only recently formed a family, but often unmarried girls still live with their parents, i.e. in senior families. The FLT-cases differ in respect of family composition: there are more children of pre-school age in these households. The FLT-cases are largely from the poorer strata of Kikuyu society; the same is true, although to a lesser extent, of the PSH participants. The trend for PSH-participants to come from poor households is actually stronger than the table indicates.[8] The difference between these two groups is that a large proportion of the FLT-cases, unlike the PSH-participants, have no land available. Quite a few of the MCH-visitors did not own land either but this can be explained by the presence of the single women and young married women in this group, who have not (yet) been given land by their father or father-in-law (Box C, p. 33).

In summary, the catchment populations of the three programmes differ considerably. Among the MCH-visitors there are relatively many young and single mothers, which probably reflects a stronger

Table 13. *Characteristics of participants in three programmes*[1]

		MCH visitors (N=656)	PSH partic. (N=152)	FLT cases (N=85)	Survey popul. (N=300)
Distance (%)					
Household-	0.1–4.9	59	93	} 37	—
centre (km)	5.0–9.9	31	} 7		—
	10.0+	10		63	—
Characteristics: mother (%)					
Age (years)	19 and below	12	1	2	2
	20–29	57	48	46	46
	30–49	32	49	50	49
	50 and over	0	1	1	2
Education	none	35	45	59	36
	standard 1–4	15	22	26	29
	standard 5–8	41	30	15	29
	secondary	10	3	0	6
Marital	single	13	4	8	3
status	married, monog.	{ 83	86	62	85
	married, polyg.	{ n.a.	4	11	7
	sep/divorced	4	5	15	2
	widow	0.5	2	4	3
Characteristics: household (%)					
Domestic	young families	38	26	26	25
stage	middle-stage	38	63	65	57
	senior families	25	11	9	18
Household size (average)		5.9	6.6	6.7	6.7
Number of	few (2 or less)	65	66	54	66
pre-school children	several (3 or more)	35	34	46	34
Income	poor household	56[2]	47	67	41
group	medium	33[2]	44	28	38
	rich	12[2]	9	5	21
Farm size	none	17	5	36	0
(acres)	0.1–0.9	13	32	13	29
	1.0–2.9	33	27	24	49
	3.0 and more	38	35	27	23

[1] An account of relevant data sources is given in Chapter 5, note 6.
[2] Percentages not comparable with figures for the other programmes, see Chapter 6, note 6.

tendency of mothers to attend with their first-born children than with later children. The PSH-participants are drawn from the poorer households, as intended, but in other respects differ little from the general population. The women admitted to FLT centres, finally, have the most specific characteristics, i.e. poverty and marital instability. They also have a lower level of education and tend to have more children of pre-school age.

The three programmes are frequented by children in a similar age range with the exception of the FLT centres where older siblings often accompany the younger child with acute problems. About one-third of the children are younger than 12 months, one-third are between 12 and 23 months and one-third are two years or older (one half in the case of the FLT programme). The nutritional condition of the children reflects the different functions of the three programmes (Table 14). The children at the FLT centres are generally in the poorest condition: they have a low to medium weight-for-height and height-for-age, which indicates not only that their present condition is poor but also that they have a poor nutrition history. The PSH-participants also show strong indications of poor previous nutrition, with a lower height-for-age than the general group of children visiting the MCH services. The PSH-children, however, generally have a positive weight-for-height, indicating that they are in a relatively stable condition (either already when they join the programme or soon after). Among the MCH-visitors, on the other hand, there are many children with a low weight-for-height and who show, at least at present, signs of distress. This accords with the fact that two-thirds of the children visited because of a health complaint, and that they must have been ill for some time, resulting in loss of weight.

Nutrition Intervention in Central Province

Table 14. *Age and nutritional status of children at different programmes*

	N	Age (months)			Average			% Children below		
		06–11 (%)	12–23 (%)	24–59 (%)	H-A (—)	W-H (—)	W-A (—)	H-A (90)	W-H (90)	W-A (80)
MCH										
Infrequent visitors	83	31	39	30	95.0	93.3	85.3	12	40	30
Frequent visitors	91	30	37	33	95.1	92.6	85.1	16	41	37
PSH										
Recent participants	93	28	37	36	93.2	97.2	86.3	25	18	22
FLT										
Cases at admission	147	18	27	55	88.7	89.6	73.3	55	47	68

Chapter 6

NIRP: Evaluation Methodology

The aim of the NIRP research project was to study the three programmes as they were actually operating, and to make the evaluation as unintrusive as possible. The organization of the programmes differed considerably and the daily management of the programmes therefore placed restraints on the evaluation, as is usual in post facto studies. It was not possible to use an identical study design in the three studies. Instead the designs were adapted to the particular conditions at each of the programmes. This chapter presents a brief description of the different constraints in each case and the designs that were finally chosen, together with a discussion of possible confounding variables. Except for some minor variations, the outcome measures or indicators are the same in each of the studies. They are discussed in the last section of this chapter.

6.1 Designs

Nutrition Field Workers

The activities of Nutrition Field Workers overlap with those of other maternal and child health (MCH) personnel and consequently it is difficult to distinguish between the activities of the Field Workers as such and those of their MCH colleagues. The focus of the evaluation therefore had to be adjusted slightly, and was ultimately defined as the nutritional effects of contact with MCH services at health centres that have Nutrition Field Workers on their staff (HN, 1980a).

Nutritional effects of contact with MCH services cannot be expected to become manifest over short periods of time, but the limited time available for data collection did not permit long observation periods. Consequently, there was no possibility of observing the same subjects before and a considerable time after the intervention. Two alternatives were considered and rejected: comparison between areas with and without health centres, and comparison between mothers with and without contact with MCH clinics. Most people in Central Province live within travelling distance of health facilities and it would have been unrealistic to look for an area where mothers had never attended MCH services. It was equally unrealistic to look for individual mothers who had never visited a MCH clinic; immunization rates are high, and people go to great lengths to find medical treatment for their children. Although mothers with first-born children are conceivably a group that has not previously been exposed, these women are generally quite young, often recently married, and thus different from the majority of mothers.

Nevertheless, people do differ in their exposure to MCH services and a comparison between frequent and infrequent visitors should, to some extent, reveal the effects of contact with MCH services and may represent a meaningful evaluation, depending on how the respective groups are selected. In the present case, visitors could not be selected from clinic records since weight charts were not handed out and no other records were kept of the visits of individual mothers and children. But even if such information had been available there would probably have been specific reasons for the more frequent attendance of certain mothers (e.g. greater motivation, higher education, illness), which would have influenced the comparison between groups. These possible confounding variables have to be controlled, and a neutral reason for difference in visits was therefore required.

It is fairly well established that attendance at MCH services depends to a large degree on the distance, or rather the time, people have to travel to reach the health centre (King, 1966; Buschkens & Slikkerveer, 1982). Long travelling times offer an understandable reason for infrequent attendance. Moreover, differences in travelling time would not in themselves influence a comparison between frequent and infrequent visitors. In view of these considerations the two following groups were finally selected for comparison: frequent visitors living nearby and infrequent visitors living far away. The frequent visitors comprised mothers [1] who had to travel less than an hour and who had visited four times or more over the past six months. The second group consisted of mothers who reported that they had to travel an hour or more and who had visited three times or less in the course of the previous half year.[2] The study was restricted to mothers bringing children between the ages of 6 and 59 months, and in cases where they were accompanied by more than one child, the child nearest to two years of age was selected as index child.[3]

This design is a variant of the post-test-only control group design, a quasi-experimental design. Since cases were not randomly selected, an additional check is required to establish whether differences of any other nature exist between the groups. In this case, further data on the two groups confirmed that there were no important social or economic differences between the frequent and infrequent visitors (HN, 1980a; 27–28). One possible objection to this design is that mothers had perhaps frequently attended over the previous half year because the child suffered from one persistent complaint. In that case selection would be the result of a particular illness of the child, and not of a general attendance pattern. This objection is, however, not confirmed by the data. The rate revisiting because of a previous complaint of the child is not significantly higher among the frequent visitors.

Pre-School Health Programme

In the case of the PSH programme a before–after design with randomization was not possible either. Again, the limited time for the study did not permit extended observation periods, in particular because the rate at which newcomers were accepted in the programme was low, no more than three or four cases a month per clinic (HN, 1980b).

The obvious alternative, a comparison between mothers with

and without contact with the programme would have been flawed because the participants in the programme come from the poorer section of the population. Any comparison with the general population would have reflected not only the effects of the programme but also other differences between the participants and the general population. Another, more suitable, alternative was to compare recent entrants with long-time participants. This type of comparison, however, is only permissible if there are no differences of a social or other nature between the mothers and children in the two groups. Such differences could arise with self-selection or selective re-attendance, i.e. if the women who drop out of the programme have characteristics which distinguish them from the other women in the programme, such as poverty or lack of interest.

A fairly simple solution to this problem was, however, possible in this study. A group of recent entrants (children admitted over the previous six months and their mothers) and a group of participants who had been attending for more than 2.5 years (1.5 years in the case of the clinic at Karaba mission) were selected and examined. In the course of the following year the clinic records were checked and the recent entrants who had stopped attending (10%) were excluded from the study. This procedure was only possible by postponing the analysis for over a year, something which is often not feasible. The group of long-time participants had frequented the PSH clinics for 33 months, on average. Inevitably, there were age differences between the children in the two groups. Further information regarding the social and economic circumstances of the participants did not indicate any important differences in characteristics that might invalidate comparison between the two groups (HN, 1980b: 30–31).

Family Life Training Centres

In the case of the two previous programmes it was not feasible to examine the same individuals before and after contact with the programme because of the long time periods that would have to be covered. The courses at the Family Life Training Centres, however, take only three weeks and this makes it possible to examine a sufficient number of mothers and children at admission and after intervention. This type of design, pre-test–post-test, requires a control group of individuals who have not been exposed to the intervention: a group that serves to establish whether changes have occurred irrespective of the intervention and, if so, to measure their magnitude (HN, 1982).

During the first half-year of 1978, 85 newly admitted mothers were interviewed at the three Family Life Training Centres in Central Province. They and each of the children that they had brought with them were seen during the first days at the centre, again shortly before they were discharged and a third time six months later at their homes. The social–economic background of these women has already been described in Chapter 4.5, where poverty and marital instability were noted as prime characteristics. The control group consisted of 100 households drawn from the larger group studied in the NIRP-survey in Murang'a District: every third household, in themselves a representative rural sample. These households were revisited after six months, and the timing of the initial survey and the revisit coincided with the interviewing at the centres and with the home-visits.[4]

The 85 cases constitute about one-third of all admissions in Central Province during that year and form a representative sample of this larger group of cases. With the exception of five early discharges, all cases were examined at admission and discharge. Of the remaining group, 61 women (with 94 children) were later located and examined at their homes. A total of 19 women (25%) could not be located and were not revisited. The latter were mostly women from young families who, although still married, already had serious marital problems at the time of admission. (In several cases this had, in fact, been one of the main reasons for admission – to give the women an opportunity to recuperate.) Six months later several of these women had indeed separated from their husbands and had left their respective homes for, at that moment, unknown destinations. By leaving their husbands women not only risk becoming homeless as described earlier, in many cases they will no longer have land available to grow their own food crops either. If they cannot fall back on relatives, they have to try to find other means of existence, but this is no easy matter. It is likely that the cases that could not be re-interviewed are a group that will face serious problems in providing a livelihood for themselves and their children in the future. Since the evaluation was limited to the cases that were examined on all three occasions, an important subgroup, probably characterized by serious social problems, was therefore excluded from the evaluation.

6.2 Non-Treatment Variables

As we have seen, there is a wide variety of social and economic differences among the Kikuyu population in Central Province, which is reflected in the different household characteristics. Many of these characteristics are interrelated and together constitute larger factors that potentially influence child nutrition and levels of nutritional status in general. What is therefore needed from the point of view of evaluation is the control of broad groups of characteristics, rather than of individual variables. Most of the differences between Kikuyu households can be understood in terms of economic resources and family composition. The three main factors of income group, domestic stage and number of young children, can be used to assess the degree of control over social and economic variables in the different studies. A summary of the household characteristics of the different groups is given in Table 15; detailed figures are listed in Appendix 4. The figures show that there are only small differences in social and economic background between the groups of frequent and infrequent MCH-visitors and the groups of recent and long-time PSH-participants. An exception is that the long-time PSH-participants more often stem from poor households than the recent participants, due to less strict criteria for admission at one of the clinics at the time (HN, 1980b). The difference, however, is small and is related to only one of the three clinics. For the present purposes it can be assumed that the groups differ only in contact with the respective programmes, and that they can therefore serve to measure the impact of the two programmes.[5] The difference in social and economic characteristics between FLT-cases and control group has already been noted in connection with the aetiology of malnutrition in Central Province (Chapter 4.6). The mutual differences between MCH-visitors, PSH-participants, FLT-cases and the general, rural population were discussed in the section on catchment populations in Chapter 5.[6]

Table 15. *Distribution of socio-economic factors in study groups*[1]

	MCH Study		PSH Study		FLT Study	
	infreq. visitors (N=83)	frequent visitors (N=91)	recent particip. (N=70)	long-time particip. (N=82)	FLT cases (N=61)	Control group (N=100)
Income group (% poor households)	61[2]	63[2]	39	55	66	42
Domestic stage (% young families)	46	37	30	23	20	24
Pre-school children (% with 3 or more p–s children)	33	33	39	30	48	35

[1] Detailed information is listed in Appendix 4.
[2] Percentages not comparable with figures for the other programmes, see Chapter 6, note 6.

6.3 Indicators

Evaluation of nutrition intervention usually relies heavily on indicators of nutritional status, but in principle indicators can be selected from various proximal as well as from more distal outcomes. Because the aim of the present studies was to gain a better insight into the influence of the interventions, different indicators were selected. They cover three levels of intervention: nutritional cognition, food consumption and nutritional status. The same measuring instruments were used in the NIRP-survey, and the various results of this survey, previously discussed, indicate that these indicators have sufficient discriminatory power. Nutritional knowledge and preferences were found to vary with educational level; food consumption and anthropometric findings varied meaningfully with other social and economic factors.

Nutritional Cognition

Interviews included several open-ended questions on nutritional knowledge. Topics included the recognition of malnutrition and the causes of kwashiorkor and marasmus. Other questions concerned the preferred duration of breastfeeding, treatment of diarrhoea, introduction age of supplementary foods[7] and required frequency of meals (Table 16). Since the answer categories are not suitable for quantitative scoring, they are difficult to aggregate. Only one composite sub-score was therefore used, consisting of the number of supplementary foods (out of four foods inquired after) that can reportedly be introduced by the age of four months or younger.

Maternal food preferences were assessed by means of a paired comparison schedule including twelve foods that differ in energy and protein content. Mothers were presented with a comparison between two foods at a time, for example between maize and beans, and asked to choose which food they would prefer to give to a two-year-old. Earlier studies had shown that this technique is well suited to measuring the maternal preferences of African rural women (Hoorweg & McDowell, 1979; HN, 1980c). Paired comparison schedules can vary according to the nature and number of stimuli (foods in the present case), but can also differ in the number of comparisons, particularly in the case of incomplete schedules. In the present case, 12 foods give a total of 66 possible comparisons. However, only 16 of the comparisons were used, i.e. the comparisons between foods that are high in energy and protein content (legumes, animal products) and foods that are high in calories but relatively low in proteins (cereals) or that are low in both calories and proteins (roots & tubers, vegetables, fruits).[8] A composite score was distilled from these comparisons, one point being added whenever a high energy/high protein food of the first category was chosen. The scores can theoretically range between 0 and 16, but in practice scores below 5 occur only incidentally. The reliability (Spearman–Brown coefficient) of the 16-item scale was calculated at .71 (HNS, 1984: 30).

Food Consumption

The food consumption of children was measured by means of a dietary recall for the previous day. Possible breast milk consumption was not measured. Mothers were asked about the foods and drinks consumed by the child in the course of the previous day and night, starting with the first dish of the day. In families where more than one child was included in the study, this information was collected for the child nearest to two years of age. The mother was requested to indicate the amounts that had been consumed with the help of a cup or plate, usually from her own household equipment. In the case of mixed dishes, they were asked to indicate the relative proportions of the major ingredients. On the basis of these proportions and with the help of average recipes collected earlier, the total weight of the cooked dish as well as the weight of the raw ingredients was estimated. The food table of Platt (1962) was used to calculate energy and protein content. A detailed description of method and calculations is given elsewhere (HNS, 1984: 30) (Box J).

Nutritional Status

The nutritional state of children was assessed by means of anthropometry. Weights were measured with Salter weighing scales in tenths of kilograms. Children were weighed without clothes except for a shirt or light jersey. All weights were later corrected for this by subtracting 150 grams. Heights were measured with a collapsible length-board with a head-rest, a detachable foot-rest and a fixed tape measure.[9] Birth dates were recorded to the day where possible. When the exact date of birth was unknown, at least the month of birth was recorded. Results for each child were compared against the Harvard standards as listed in Jelliffe (1966), and three indices were computed. Height-for-age (H-A) expresses the height of the child as a percentage of the standard height expected for the age of the child. Weight-for-height (W-H) converts the weight of the child into a percentage of the standard weight expected for the height of the child. Weight-for-age (W-A) does not allow for height and expresses the weight of the child as a percentage of the standard weight for the age of the child.

These three indices reflect different although not altogether independent aspects of nutritional status (Waterlow, 1976; Keller, 1983). If a child is not adequately nourished its weight gain slows down and it may even start to lose weight. The child becomes wasted and shows a low weight-for-height. Length growth will also slow down if this situation persists and in the long run the child may become stunted and show a low height-for-age. When nutrition improves the weight of the child may recover rapidly until it reaches the weight corresponding to its height. Height growth may also respond, but more slowly and the losses suffered are often not compensated for. Height-for-age, therefore, reflects the nutritional history of the child and a low height-for-age (stunting) indicates an inadequate intake relative to need over long duration, i.e. the possible chronicity of malnutrition. In contrast, weight-for-height reveals transitory variations in the condition of the child and a low weight-for-height (wasting) reveals acute distress. The meaning of these two measures, therefore, differs with age: weight-for-height is the most significant measure among very young children, height-for-age becomes more significant with age. Weight-for-age presents a combined index of nutritional state; a low weight-for-age often reflects a combination of wasting and stunting, and it is a useful measure for groups of mixed age composition.

Owing to differences in conditions between the programmes and differences in study designs it was not always possible to collect full information on each of the outcome measures. Appendix 4 lists the information that was collected in each of the study

***Box J.* The measurement of food consumption**

Dietary recall and dietary record (observation) are the methods most commonly used to study food consumption. The dietary recall, as described in the text, is an interview method that estimates food intake of the previous day with the help of the recollection of the respondents. The dietary record, on the other hand, measures and weighs food consumption as it takes place. A number of studies, mostly in Western countries, have compared results of the two different methods. The general conclusion from these studies is that there is reasonable agreement between overall, group-wise results but that there is far less agreement between estimates of individual consumption. As regards the recall method, some authors mention a tendency of respondents to over-estimate small quantities and under-report large quantities. Such a regression effect purportedly has no influence on group averages but would reduce variation in general: the flat-slope syndrome. As regards dietary records it has been suggested that respondents tend to serve their 'best' and 'favourite' dishes on such days, resulting in various misrepresentations (Block, 1982).

During the NIRP-survey, observations on food consumption were recorded in a sub-sample of 100 cases, in addition to the recall schedule for the previous day. The time period covered by the two methods therefore was not the same, although of the same duration. Table J1 lists the frequency of consumption of dishes according to the different methods; Table J2 the size of the daily portions consumed.

Table J1. *Children consuming dishes (%)*

	Dietary record	Dietary recall[1]
Githeri	69	48
Gitoero	29	44
Ucuru	28	26
Ngima	36	58
Rice	4	2
Roots, single	38	26
Stew	15	22
Tea	68	76
Milk, single	43	67
Miscellaneous	36	35

[1] Previous day

The comparison reveals that both recall and observation methods suffer from inaccuracies. When under observation women tended to prepare more of the favourite dishes. This is shown by a more frequent consumption of githeri and accompanying changes in the consumption of other dishes. Gitoero and ngima were eaten less often, but single roots more often, usually in addition to githeri. The recall method, on the other hand, though probably reflecting the usual composition of the diet more accurately tends to overestimate the daily portions of certain dishes, such as stew and roots eaten single, and also the frequency of milk consumption. The resulting errors, however, are not of such a magnitude that the estimates of protein and energy consumption are seriously distorted (energy consumption may be overestimated by 5% or less) (HNS, 1984: 74).

Table J2. *Average daily portions for children consuming dishes (grams)[2]*

	Dietary record	Dietary recall[1]
Githeri	358 (243)	333 (184)
Gitoero	358 (299)	325 (170)
Ucuru	426 (206)	420 (235)
Ngima	281 (129)	292 (160)
Rice	n.a.	n.a.
Roots, single	220 (133)	334 (222)
Stew	121 (43)	157 (88)
Tea	590 (363)	569 (285)
Milk, single	357 (219)	382 (240)
Miscellaneous	112 (78)	114 (88)

[1] Previous day
[2] Standard deviation in parenthesis
Source: HNS, 1984: 71

In addition to the average sizes of the daily portions, Table J2 also lists standard deviations. The flat-slope syndrome, if present, should lead to lesser variation among the recall data. Although it is true that for three dishes the (recall) standard deviations are considerably smaller, this is not sufficient evidence of a general reduction in variance as a result of the recall method.

conditions.[10] It may be noted that among the FLT-cases food consumption was recorded only during the home visit. Furthermore, that among the MCH-visitors a partial knowledge questionnaire was included and that among the control group nutritional knowledge was examined during the first visit only.

Chapter 7

The Impact of the Programmes

7.1 Nutritional Cognition

In general, nutritional awareness among rural Kikuyu women is neither extremely low nor high. Usually, 40–60% of the women answered questions on nutrition correctly (Table 16). In general the newcomers to the three programmes (infrequent MCH-visitors, recent PSH-participants, FLT-cases at admission) did not do any worse than mothers in the control group with the exception of the question of diarrhoea. Diarrhoea often plays a crucial role in causing malnutrition and Oral Rehydration Therapy was only starting to be advised at the time. PSH-participants and FLT-cases seem to be far less knowledgeable about the treatment of diarrhoea. Noteworthy is the high nutritional awareness of mothers who are admitted to FLT centres. On virtually all questions these women give a higher percentage of correct answers than respondents in the other programmes and even than women in the general population. It seems unlikely that this high level of knowledge and preferences is a true characteristic of this group. It is more probable that during the illness of the child and, as a result of contacts with neighbours and health personnel, the women have somehow become sensitized to the nutritional needs of children. Although

Table 16. Nutritional knowledge of mothers in different study groups

	MCH study		PSH study			FLT study		
	infreq. visitors (N=83)	frequent visitors (N=91)	recent particip. (N=70)	long-time particip. (N=82)	admission (N=61)	dis-charge (N=61)	home visit (N=61)	control group (N=100)
Recognition and causation of malnutrition								
1. Recognition kwashiorkor (%)	—	—	89	98	92	95	85	98
2. Causation kwashiorkor (%)	—	—	53	61	66	71	69	60
3. Causation marasmus (%)	59	48	48	56	59	67	59	43
Supplementary foods and breastfeeding								
4. Number of foods introduced by 4 months of age (average)[1]	1.0	1.4	1.2	2.0	2.2	2.0	1.9	1.0
5. Prefer to wean at 14 months or earlier (%)	35	39	37	52	34	40	38	45
Food requirements								
6. Regard more than 3 feedings a day necessary (%)	—	—	49	43	67	61	53	41
7. Treat diarrhoea with water with sugar or salt (%)	25	30	14	9	15	13	10	42

[1] Out of 4 foods inquired after, see p. 97

the level of their earlier nutritional knowledge is not known, the findings nevertheless suggest that ignorance does not play a major role in the occurrence of malnutrition. Regarding improvements in nutritional cognition, neither of the programmes achieves spectacular results. Only the PSH programme shows a slight influence on nutritional knowledge, but increases in the percentage of correct answers at best reach 15% and are rarely significant (Table 16).

MCH. In the case of the intervention by Nutrition Field Workers, few increases in knowledge are observed except for an earlier introduction of supplementary foods.[1]

PSH. In the case of the PSH programme, some minor improvements can be noted regarding the recognition and causation of malnutrition. Larger differences occur regarding the introduction age of supplementary foods and the duration of breastfeeding. Mothers who have participated for a long time show a tendency to introduce foods at an earlier age, a trend which may be appreciated positively. However, there are also some changes in the preferred duration of breastfeeding. Long-time participants more often find it advisable to wean before 14 months, which would be an understandable, although unintended, side-effect of the attention in nutrition instruction for foods other than breastmilk. This suggests that there is a trend to discontinue the traditional practice of prolonged breastfeeding, although it must be pointed out that few women feel that children should be weaned very early, before nine months. (A similar trend was noted on detailed examination of the data on MCH-visitors.[2])

FLT. The effects of the FLT programme on nutritional cognition are also small. Although some minor increases are noted at discharge from the centres, these improvements have largely disappeared after six months. In fact, knowledge at admission and at the time of the home visit is nearly identical, except for two topics on which a decline in awareness may be observed. These are the introduction age of supplementary foods and the required frequency of feeding – the two points on which the FLT-cases had shown themselves to be most sensitized at admission, and it appears that after this period of six months there is a return to normal levels of awareness.

Table 17. *Maternal preferences for high energy/high protein foods*[1] *(averages and standard deviations)*

MCH study		PSH study		FLT study		
infreq. visitors (N=83)	frequent visitors (N=91)	recent particip. (N=70)	long-time particip. (N=82)	admission (N=61)	home visit (N=61)	control group (N=100)
11.5 (2.4)	11.5 (2.9)	11.4 (2.6)	12.3 (2.4)	12.5 (2.1)	13.1 (1.9)	10.4 (2.6)

[1] Number of choices for legumes and animal products (maximum score: 16).

The trends in nutritional preferences prove to be more or less similar (Table 17). The three groups of newcomers all report a somewhat higher preference for legumes and animal products than the general population. This suggests that the FLT-cases were not the only group to be sensitized at admission, but that MCH- and PSH-newcomers also tended to give more positive answers. Among the MCH-visitors and FLT-cases there are no indications of any effects as a result of exposure to the programmes.[3] The only significant shift in preferences occurs between recent and long-time participants of the PSH programme.[4] This difference results from an increase in choices for peas, eggs and meat, fewer choices for roots & tubers, while the choices for cereals and vegetables remained constant. That the PSH programme is the only form of intervention that influences nutritional preferences accords with the finding that it was also the only programme to exert a certain influence on nutritional knowledge.

7.2 Food Consumption

Food consumption as indicator of nutritional change does not lend itself easily to comparison across programmes because of differences in age composition between the groups of children selected in the three studies.[5] The presentation in this section is, therefore, restricted to children who were no longer breastfed and who were between the ages of 6 and 35 months.

MCH. Table 18 shows that there is little difference in food intake between the children in the two MCH groups. Energy and protein intake are much the same and the composition of energy intake is also virtually identical. The contribution of cereals, milk, roots & tubers, and legumes is about 35%, 25%, 15% and 7% respectively in both groups. There are no signs that the diets of the children of frequent visitors have been influenced by contact with the Nutrition Field Workers at the health centres.

Table 18. *MCH Study: Summary of food consumption (age group 6–35 months, not breastfed)*

	Infrequent visitors (N=42)	Frequent visitors (N=53)
Average (standard dev.)		
Energy (kcal.)	785 (375)	785 (359)
Protein (g.)	29 (18)	25 (15)
Contribution to energy intake (%)		
Cereals	34	37
Milk	24	25
Roots & tubers	16	16
Legumes	8	6
Other	18	16

PSH. No difference in energy and protein intake was found to exist between children of recent and children of long-time participants (Table 19). The composition of the daily energy intake was also very similar, with the possible exception of milk consumption which seems slightly lower among the long-time participants. Since mothers were interviewed during their monthly visit to the clinic it can be assumed that the food rations of the previous month had, by and large, been exhausted. The diet at this particular point in time therefore indicates what mothers feed their children when restricted to their own resources: i.e. any possible changes that occur in maternal behaviour. No discernible influence in this respect was observed, although of course, the food rations themselves are not taken into account here.

FLT. In the case of the FLT study, the dietary recall was recorded during the home visit only, so that comparison with diets before admission to the centre was not possible.[6] Table 20 shows that,

Table 19. *PSH Study: Summary of food consumption (age group 6–35 months, not breastfed)*

	Recent particip. (N=37)	Long-time particip. (N=27)
Average (standard dev.)		
Energy (kcal.)	886 (373)	908 (343)
Protein (g.)	31 (16)	33 (22)
Contribution to energy intake (%)		
Cereals	45	44
Milk	16	12
Roots & tubers	16	12
Legumes	12	15
Other	11	17

six months after discharge, the energy intake of the FLT-cases in the 6–35 months age range, is considerably lower than that of the control group. On the one hand this is understandable because the FLT-children generally come from poor households where food consumption is lower. On the other hand it means that the nutrition instruction has not succeeded sufficiently in increasing the food allocation to the child and that, after intervention, a lag in the food intake of FLT-children continues to exist. Not only do they eat less, they also eat differently, they consume relatively less milk and less roots & tubers.

Table 20. *FLT Study: Summary of food consumption (age group 6–35 months, not breastfed)*

	FLT cases (N=42)	Control group (N=48)
Average (standard dev.)		
Energy (kcal.)	1095 (407)	1257 (341)
Protein (g.)	42 (20)	40 (15)
Contribution to energy intake (%)		
Cereals	50	38
Milk	18	25
Roots & tubers	7	20
Legumes	13	8
Other	12	9

7.3 Nutritional Status

The nutritional status of the different groups at admission has already been discussed in Chapter 5.4. The children visiting the MCH centres have a lower W-H (weight-for-height) than the PSH-participants, reflecting conditions of acute distress. The PSH-participants in turn have a lower H-A (height-for-age), which reflects a poorer nutritional history. The FLT group with many severely malnourished children generally has a lower W-H and H-A than the two other groups.

MCH. The condition of the children of frequent MCH-visitors is shown in Table 21. The different indicators, H-A, W-H and W-A, are not noticeably better in this group than among the infrequent visitors. The percentage of children showing symptoms of acute distress (low W-H) is more or less the same, indicating that the children in the two groups were probably brought to the centres for similar health complaints. Height-for-age, the most telling indicator of long-term nutritional status is also the same in the two

Table 21. *MCH Study: Summary of nutritional status (children, aged 6–59 months)*

	N	Average H-A	W-H	W-A	Percentage below H-A (90)	W-H (90)	W-A (80)
Infrequent visitors	83	95.0 (5.6)	93.3 (9.0)	85.3 (11.6)	12	40	30
Frequent visitors	91	95.1 (5.1)	92.6 (9.9)	85.1 (12.9)	16	41	37

groups, while the percentage of children below the critical value of W-A (80) is, finally, not any lower among the frequent visitors. Thus there are no indications of a positive influence on nutritional status as a result of contact with Nutrition Field Workers at the health centres.

PSH. Comparison of the nutritional status of the recent and long-time participants was hampered in two ways. Firstly, there is a considerable age difference between the children in the two groups

(Table 22). Secondly, clinic records show that 2.5 years ago, over 40% of the participants joining the programme were below W-A (80), while of the recent admissions only 17% fell below this weight criterion. It is likely that the cause of the poorer condition of children at that time lies in the relative drought conditions which occurred during the period 1974–75 and which necessitated food relief in various parts of the country.[7] It is not clear whether this difference reflects lower weights, lower heights or a combination of both because the height of children was not routinely recorded at the centres. This makes any further comparison between the two groups difficult.

Table 22. *PSH Study: Summary of nutritional status (children aged 6–59 months)*

	N	Average W-A	% below W-A (80)
Long-time participants			
At admission[1]	93	80.2 (13.9)	44
At time of study[2]	93	83.4 (9.2)	41
Recent participants			
At admission[3]	88	87.2 (11.5)	17

[1] 1973–1976
[2] 1978
[3] 1977–1978

Analysis therefore concentrated on the progress of long-time participants as such. Comparison of this group at admission, in 1973–76, and at the time of study in 1978 shows that only little change in W-A has occurred, that no catch-up growth has occurred and that the condition of the children has remained more or less the same. However, a comparison of W-A is not sufficient to ascertain whether any changes in nutritional status have occurred. For example, it is possible for W-H levels to improve while H-A lags further behind. In such cases average W-A would hardly change, despite important changes in nutritional condition.

Further insight was gained from an analysis of the weight progress of the long-time participants according to age at admission to the programmes, and as recorded by the clinic staff.[8] This analysis reveals that the older the children are on admission, the poorer their overall condition is likely to be (Figure 10). This is

Figure 10. *Weight progress of long-time PSH participants
(listed are the average weight-for-age of groups of children admitted at
different ages, after having participated in the programme for different
periods of time)*

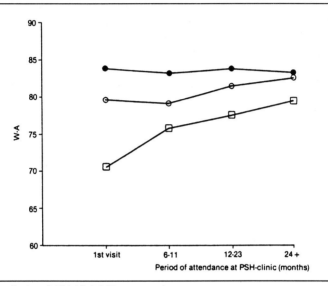

Key (age of child at first visit to programme):

—●— below 1 year (N = 44)   —⊖— 1 year old (N = 26)   —⊟— 2 years and older (N = 13)

Source: HN, 1980b: 38, 39, 49

quite understandable in view of what is known about the growth
and development of Kikuyu children. Children generally show a
decline in W-H after the first year of age, particularly children
from poor households (like many PSH participants) and children
in the 12–35 months age range: a decline which is accompanied
by stunting of various degrees. Although the children joining the
programme at a later age are generally in a poorer condition at
admission, they show more compensation in weight: a considerable
compensation in the case of children over two years old. Nevertheless, on average, the two older age groups still remain below

111

the H-A level of the younger age group as measured at the time of examination (H-A = 92.0, 91.0, and 90.4 in order of admission age). Apparently, late entrants to the programme have suffered growth faltering that is not or only partially compensated for. In this context it is significant that children entering the programme at an *early* stage, i.e. before one year of age, generally continue to grow at the weight level at which they entered and that they do not show the expected further decline in weight. Since the cases have similarly disadvantaged backgrounds it is likely that the height level of the younger entrants would have declined to the same extent as that of the older entrants if they had not participated in the programme. The indications therefore are that children continue to grow at the level at which they join the programme, which can be considered a modest but nevertheless important result. In fact, it is the goal as formulated in the programme objectives: to maintain the growth of children at their potential level.

FLT. The programme generally deals with severe cases of malnutrition, although not all children who are admitted are necessarily severely malnourished: 70% fall below W-A (80) and 14% below W-A (60).[9] The first question is whether there is a high mortality among this group. Slightly over 100 children were examined at admission to the centres. One child died shortly afterwards at the centre. All of the remaining children were found present during the home visit some six months later, except for two children who were reportedly absent, although the possibility exists that one of these children had died. In Kenya, the mortality rate of children between the ages of one and four is around 20 per 1000, or 1 per 100 over a period of six months. With one or possibly two deaths in a period of six months in this case, there is no indication of an unusual mortality among the FLT-cases.

The condition at admission varies between different age groups (Table 23). In the youngest group many cases show signs of acute distress and fall below W-H (85). In the older age groups the degree of stunting is much higher. It is probably because of this that the different age groups react quite differently to the treatment at the centres. The weight gains of the younger groups are smaller than those of the older age groups. Under normal conditions young children tend to gain weight more rapidly than older children, but many of the young children show no weight increase at all during their stay at the centre. The very youngest group, in fact, gains so little weight that their daily weight increase is lower than that of children of the same age in a control group. Apparently very young children, who are often still breastfed, are difficult to treat and do not react quickly to the regimen at the centre. The older children, although more stunted, are otherwise probably in stable condition and appear to profit more directly from their stay at the centres (Box K).

The long-term gains over a period of six months, however, show a somewhat different pattern (Figures 11, 12). Weight and height growth of the children in the two youngest age groups are nearly

Table 23. *FLT Study: Summary of nutritional status by age group*

	Age (months)			
	06–11 (N=18)	12–23 (N=24)	24–35 (N=21)	36–59 (N=31)
Condition at admission				
Children below W-H (85) (%)	33	42	24	0
Children below H-A (90) (%)	22	58	76	68
Recovery at centre				
Weight increase (g/day)	4.7	10.2	12.3	22.1
Children without weight increase (%)	39	29	29	19

the same as that of their peers in a control group. This means that the condition of the (young) cases does not deteriorate any further, contrary to what is suggested by the previous findings during the stay at the centre. However, there are no signs of improvement or catch-up growth.

The two-year-old children show a lesser weight[10] and height[11] growth than control children during the six months between admission and home visit (although the latter difference is not statistically significant). This means that the relative nutritional status of these children has deteriorated even further during this period. Why this age group shows such lack of progress and such different results from the other groups is not clear.

The weight spurt of the eldest group (aged three to four years) slows down after discharge. Over the total period of six months they show the same weight progress as a group of control children. However, they do show significantly greater height gains than the control group over this period and achieve a certain degree of

113

Box K. **Progress of wasted children**

Nutrition rehabilitation aims particularly at the convalescence of severely malnourished children, although siblings are also admitted to the FLT centres. The intervention is designed to improve the condition of children in a short period of time. It was already described how older children who are in relatively stable condition manage to realize greater (relative) weight increases than the younger children, who are more often in condition of acute distress. In Table K1 this is analyzed in more detail with the help of a comparison between the growth rates of FLT-children below W-H (85), children above W-H (85) and the growth rates of control children. The difference in weight gain at the centres between the groups of wasted children and other FLT-children are small. Over the long term, however, there are differences in growth patterns. The figures demonstrate that the wasted children first recover weight while height growth remains behind. The growth effort of these children goes into weight increase which results in improvements in weight-for-height. The other group of children, on the other hand, do increase more in height, realizing a certain degree of catch-up growth.

Table K1. *Weight and height growth of FLT-cases*

	N	At Centre g/day	6-month period g/day	cm/year
W-H < 85	21	13.1 (+6.3)[1]	8.3 (+1.5)	8.0 (−0.8)
W-H > 85	73	13.7 (+8.1)	5.1 (−0.5)	8.7 (+1.0)

[1] The figures in parentheses present the deviation of the observed values from the values of the control group corrected for age differences.

Although the wasted children as a group show weight progress this does not mean that each individual child improves. There were 21 children with W-H below 85. Of this group, eight children showed a low weight increase while at the centre, and seven children had a long-term weight increase that was less than that of control children of the same age (Table K2). The latter two groups consisted mostly of the same children, six children had neither satisfactory gains at the centres, nor over the longer period of six months. Apparently, among wasted children lack of weight gain at the centres strongly predicts lack of long-term progress as well.

Table K2. *Weight gains of wasted children (W-H <85)*

		Long-term gains[2] Below age rate	Above age rate
Short-term gains[1]	Below age rate	6	2
	Above age rate	1	12

[1] Weight gains at FLT centre
[2] Weight gains over 6-months period
Source: HN, 1982: 33

catch-up growth.[12] It is plausible to relate this growth spurt to the fact that these children had gained relatively much weight at the centres, at a time when they were otherwise in stable condition.

Figure 11. *Progress of children admitted to FLT centres (average weight gain over period of 6 months)*

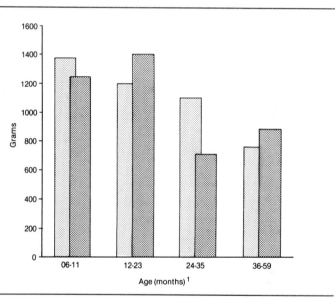

[1]Information on group composition is listed in Appendix 4.

Key: ▧ Control group ▨ FLT children

Source: HN, 1982:46

7.4 Interaction Between Intervention and Environment

Targeted or selective nutrition intervention starts from the assumption that certain groups of the population are more in need of assistance than others. A first aspect that requires scrutiny, is whether the intervention indeed succeeds in reaching those target groups, to the exclusion of other groups. The three programmes are moderately successful in this respect, as already discussed. Because interventions often aim to correct particular deficits, the further – usually implicit – assumption is that a particular intervention will be more successful among the particular group it aims at than among other groups. Nutrition education aims to compensate deficits in nutritional cognition, and should achieve most effect in situations where ignorance plays an important role in the causation of malnutrition. Supplementation aims to alleviate shortages at household level, and might therefore be expected to achieve most effects in deficit situations, i.e. among poor households and in marginal areas. Nutrition rehabilitation generally concentrates on severely malnourished children who, as we know, often come from poor households. In terms of evaluation, this translates into the question whether participants from target groups benefit more than others from contact with the programmes.

Figure 12. *Progress of children admitted to FLT centres (average height gain over period of 6 months)*

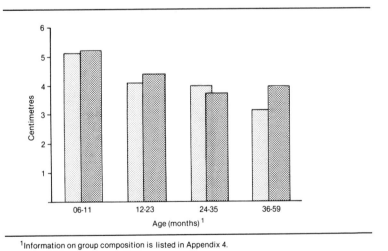

[1]Information on group composition is listed in Appendix 4.

Key: ☐ Control group ▨ FLT children

Source: HN, 1982:46

In more concrete terms this entails analysis of interaction effects, i.e. whether in certain sub-conditions or among certain subgroups effects are greater than in other conditions or groups. Because of limitations due to the number of cases that were examined at the different programmes the analysis in our case is limited to only two environmental factors: ecological area and income group. Ecological conditions were initially expected to be of major importance since they determine important variations in living conditions. However, in Central Province, households appear able to adapt to different ecological conditions in various ways so that only minor differences in nutritional conditions occur. In fact, as shown earlier, differences in available economic resources between households influence nutrition and nutritional status more strongly.

The discussion of interaction, here, is limited to differences in the nutritional status of the children and is not concerned with nutritional cognition and food consumption. Ignorance does not play a major role in the causation of malnutrition in this region of Kenya, while none of the programmes was particularly successful in improving nutritional cognition.[13] Furthermore, the restrictions in age composition of the groups of children for which information on food consumption was compared hinder interaction analysis.

MCH. The target group of the Nutrition Field Workers are young (pre-school) children in general and, as noted, there were no indications of differences in nutritional status between the groups of frequent and infrequent visitors. Not surprisingly, a breakdown of data by area and income group does not result in any differences either (Table 24).

Table 24. *MCH Study: Height-for-age by area and income group (average)*

	N	Total (s.d.)	Area			Income group	
			lower	middle	upper	poor	med./rich
Infrequent visitors	83	95.0 (5.6)	94.1	95.9	94.8	94.4	95.9
Frequent visitors	91	95.1 (5.1)	95.3	95.5	94.5	94.1	97.0

PSH. The target group in the case of the PSH programme are the needy households and, as shown, the programme manages to concentrate largely on this group. Table 25 lists the W-A results broken down by ecological area and income group. There are

117

indications that children in the lower, marginal, area improve more than those in other areas, their average W-A rising from 75.9 to 84.1. However, this particular group was older in age when admitted than the groups in the other areas, and they were also in poorest condition at that time. The greater increase in weight of this group is thus – if only partly – accounted for by the aforementioned trend that late entrants are generally in poorer condition and subsequently show greater weight increase.

Table 25. *PSH Study: Weight-for-age by area and income group (average)*

	N	Total (s.d.)	Area lower	Area middle	Area upper	Income group poor	Income group med./rich
Long-time participants							
At admission	75	80.2 (13.9)	75.9	79.1	85.6	81.5	78.6
At time of study	75	82.9 (9.2)	84.1	82.1	83.1	81.8	84.5

Results by income group run counter to the hypothesis that children in needy families will benefit most. Whereas the condition of children from poor households has remained at the same level, the condition of children from medium and rich households has improved substantially. That food supplementation is perhaps more successful where the lack of resources is least pronounced might be because in the latter case the food supplement is less likely to be shared with household members and more likely to reach the target child. However, it must be mentioned that the two trends noted are to a large extent caused by the same children, and are therefore partially identical.

FLT. Since FLT-children are sent home after a short period of rehabilitation and the families further left to their own devices, families in more favourable circumstances might be expected to be able to sustain higher growth rates in the long term. This proves not the case (Table 26). The differences between the income groups in respect of weight and height gains over the period of six months are small, and there is no suggestion that the children from medium and rich households in the long run are able to profit more from the treatment. The same applies in respect of ecological area, with one exception. Children in the middle area gain relatively more weight, but less height than the children in the two

other centres. This trend, however, can be explained by the fact
that the children at the middle centre generally had lower weight-
for-height at admission.

In all, there is little evidence of interaction effects[14] and there
are no indications that any of the programmes are particularly

Table 26. *FLT Study: Weight and height growth by area and
income group (period between admission and home visit)*

	Total (s.d) (N=94)	Area lower (N=31)	middle (N=27)	upper (N=36)	Income group poor (N=62)	med./rich (N=32)
Weight (g/day)	5.8 (4.7)	5.3	6.9	5.5	6.0	5.5
Height (cm/year)	8.5 (4.1)	9.1	7.9	8.4	8.9	7.8

successful with certain target groups. However, some reservations
should be made here. The programmes operate among selected
cases which are in need of their services, and consequently we
know little about the kind of effects that the interventions
would have had among healthy children from normal households.
Secondly, although the present studies were initially designed to
investigate possible interaction effects, the actual designs that were
finally employed had to be adapted to the daily operations of the
programmes. It was not possible to carry out sensitive tests of
interaction as a direct limitation of the quasi-experimental research
methods that were employed. At the same time it can also be said
that any existing interaction effects were apparently not strong
enough to overcome this handicap.

Chapter 8

Conclusion

8.1 Child Nutrition in Central Province

Many if not most social–economic differences between rural Kikuyu households can be understood in terms of income group and family composition. The division into income groups employed here is based on commercial farming and employment outside the farm. Poor households have neither source of income and depend on whatever income is derived from day-labour of husband and wife and what they are able to grow on their usually modest farm. Poor households not only have a smaller share in the money economy but also have less subsistence potential. Among the general population, 40% of the households sampled had to be qualified as poor, and of these households three out of four reported that they were not able to grow enough food to feed the members of the household.

Family composition is reflected mainly in domestic stage and family size. The striking thing about present-day Kikuyu life is the degree to which the nuclear family predominates. Few families have a composition other than husband, wife and children, while half the families live on their own compound by the time they have reached senior stage. The importance of the nuclear family as the basic unit of Kikuyu social structure is also reflected in the limited amount of outside support that housewives receive with their domestic tasks. The main source of assistance are the older or grown-up children. Consequently, in cases where several young children follow closely on each other mothers often find it difficult to cope with the daily household chores without the assistance of grown-up children.

In general Kikuyu mothers are reasonably familiar with important principles of child nutrition. They are generally able to recognize malnutrition and are aware of its nutritional causes. Most mothers breastfeed their children at least until the age of one, nearly all introduce various supplementary foods quite early. This is not to say that there is no room for improvement in nutritional knowledge. The understanding of the precise causes of malnutrition is often incomplete while the need of multiple feedings could be recognized more widely. Nevertheless there is no evidence of a serious lack of nutritional knowledge or of detrimental weaning practices.

Kikuyu children, in fact, have a fairly varied diet. Consumption of milk is remarkably high, taken alone or together with tea, and dairy farming is evidently of great importance for child nutrition in this region of Kenya. Roots, tubers and starchy fruits also contribute a major part of the diet. With age the consumption of these items decreases while the consumption of cereals increases. Almost half the amount of cereals consumed consists of maize flour. None the less, maize flour is not nearly as predominant an item in the daily diet as is generally assumed, while only very small amounts of sorghum and finger millet are eaten by young children. There is a general trend among Kikuyu children of satisfactory protein intake, but of a relative decrease in energy intake with age. Protein consumption is high in all age groups. Energy intake among one- and two-year-olds is also above internationally accepted standards. But among the three- to four-year-olds the average amounts of energy per kg body weight fall below FAO requirements. Energy intake is constituted mainly by four food groups: roots, tubers and starchy fruits; cereals; milk; and legumes. The latter three food groups also account for most protein intake.

In general the nutritional state of young children in Central Province compares rather favourably with that of children in other parts of Kenya, and even more so when compared with children in other tropical countries. Mean height-for-age is 93, mean weight-for-height is 96, and mean weight-for-age is 86. Based on a cross-classification of W-H and H-A, at least 60% of the children can be considered as being in normal condition. However, there is considerable variation among households; a sizeable group of children, 20–30%, show signs of malnutrition and under certain social and economic conditions high-risk situations exist. The number of children falling below W-H (90) is roughly 20%, the same percentage falls under H-A (90). Almost 30% of children had a W-A below 80, and just over 1% of the children were under W-A (60).

Formal education generally has a positive relation with nutritional cognition. Mothers with some years of secondary education are more aware of the general principles of child nutrition and have more positive nutritional preferences. Although they tend to stop breastfeeding somewhat earlier, they also tend to wait a bit longer before introducing children to the full adult diet. However, no relation was found between educational level of the mothers and food consumption of children, indicating that actual intake is probably more likely to be determined by prevailing cultural patterns and the availability of resources.

Food consumption is related to income group, and the favourable findings on intake levels do not apply to children from poor households. Energy intake of children from poor and medium households lags considerably behind that of children from rich households, and this is particularly so among the children at the vulnerable age of one year. At that age the differences in average energy intake between children from different income groups range from 200 to 400 kcal., differences which are mostly the result of a lower consumption of milk and cereals. Other household characteristics regarding family composition are not related with differences in energy intake.

Variations in ecology relate to population density and social–economic characteristics such as farm size, type of commercial farming and type of food crops cultivated. Despite differences in agricultural potential, however, households in different ecological zones appear to be in rather similar economic circumstances due to lower population densities and the accommodating role of employment in town. Consequently, there is little difference in food consumption and nutritional status between the children in different ecological areas. There are, however, signs of rapid seasonal fluctuations in weight with a drop in weight during the dry season, the lowest weight levels probably being reached shortly before the long-rain harvests.

Of all variables studied, income group shows the strongest relation with the nutritional state of young children. Furthermore, children from crowded households, that is with three or more children under six, also show lower height levels. A particularly grave situation exists where these two factors occur together, in poor households with several children of pre-school age. At the end of the dry season over 60% of the young children in these households were below W-A (80) compared with only 20% among the rest of the child population.

The relation between income group and nutritional faltering appears to be quite straightforward. Fewer available resources result in a lower energy intake among young children, particularly during the second year of life, which in turn leads to nutritional stunting. The pressure of several young children in the household, however, which is also connected with lower nutritional status, was not related to lower food consumption, as measured here, and an explanation for this may possibly be sought in differences in the quality of child care, which may lead to more insidious differences in nutrition and child development.

In an earlier monograph the general need for selective intervention was argued, what is now called targeting (Hoorweg & McDowell, 1979). In this respect, the situation is no different in Central Province. The aetiology of malnutrition in this part of Kenya is connected with pressure on economic resources and peer pressure within families, unlike the situation in other parts of Africa (and Kenya) where a relation has often been noted between malnutrition and ignorance, detrimental weaning practices and poor diets. A separate factor is marital instability, although in this case lack of resources and lack of maternal attention probably operate in combination because of the living conditions of many divorced women. None of these factors shows any indications of positive developments in the near future. With the rapidly growing population of Central Province there will be increasing pressure on the land and it is foreseeable that more households will fall below the poverty line, with the accompanying nutritional consequences. Since the crowding of young children forms one of the at-risk conditions this indicates the importance of child spacing, but the birth rates for Central Province are no different from the (high) rate of Kenya in general. There are no indications that divorce rates are slowing down; on the contrary, complex legal and social changes affect family life without, as yet, sufficient improvements in the economic position of women.

These findings underscore the need to target nutrition intervention programmes and to take into account the special needs of certain groups. In the poor households it is particularly the children in the age group of 6–23 months (not breastfed) who are at risk. The findings also indicate how the diet of young children from such households can be improved and the elements that need to be stressed in nutrition education. Preferably, children should be given more milk to drink and at the same time be given more maize flour in the form of ucuru or ngima. This has the advantage of increasing palatability without loss of energy density. When milk is not available and cannot be purchased either, mothers should be advised to rely more on legumes, something which they are likely to do anyway as the children get older. It is furthermore evident that, in addition to nutritional instruction and the treatment of acutely malnourished children, there is also a need for food supplementation programmes in Central Province under the existing conditions of intensive land use and limited employment opportunities.

8.2 Nutrition Intervention

This monograph is concerned with programmes representing the three major types of nutrition intervention existing in Kenya, variants of which are found in many countries in Africa and Asia: nutrition education, food supplementation and nutrition rehabilitation. Each of the three programmes studied appears to have a constituency of its own, with its own characteristics, although selection does not go so far that the programmes cater for completely different groups.

Nutrition instruction is given by Nutrition Field Workers who are part of the MCH teams at rural health centres. This kind of intervention appeared to have little or no impact on the nutritional attitudes or behaviour of mothers nor on the nutritional status of children. Only minor improvements in nutritional knowledge could be credited to frequent contact with the MCH services. It has to be seriously questioned whether nutrition instruction in this kind of setting can really be expected to influence parental behaviour and consequently child nutrition. In retrospect it is hardly surprising that this expectation is not met. Many of the children brought to the centres are ill. The audience is usually quite crowded and noisy, with a lot of distractions, while the instructors usually have to address a group whose individual needs are unknown to them. On the other hand, when dealing with mothers individually, health workers are often hampered by lack of case information due to the kind of records that are kept. The general conclusion must be that this kind of instruction can only offer a minor contribution to nutritional improvements and can, at best, foster the gradual spread of nutritional knowledge over longer periods of time. (In which case, it should be remembered, it is extremely difficult to evaluate such improvements, because they become impossible to distinguish from general changes among the population). There are indeed indications that this has been happening over the past decades. The general level of nutritional knowledge among women in Central Province, compared with early reports, suggests that progress has been made (Paterson, 1943). But it is likely that other factors, notably generally rising levels of education and mass communication, have had considerable impact as well, although the relative importance of these factors is hard to evaluate.

The second type of intervention under study was food supplementation. Like most supplementation programmes, the Pre-School Health Programme combines two forms of intervention: distribution of supplementary food rations on the one hand, and nutrition instruction with monthly weight monitoring on the other. The main reason why mothers are willing to attend every month is, of course, the distribution of food rations. The time and effort needed to travel every month to the distribution centre and the many waiting hours are in themselves an investment in time. For this reason alone, one would expect women with relatively sufficient resources to show little interest in joining the programme and, in fact, the findings confirm that the programme mainly reaches the poorer sections of the population. This contradicts the criticism that the small fees charged at the PSH clinics exclude participation by poor households. (Although it is likely that very poor mothers can indeed not afford to join the programme, particularly if they wish to bring more than one child).

Knowledge and preferences of the mothers did show some

improvements although the general level of nutritional knowledge among long-time participants still left considerable room for improvement. The educational effort, however, appeared to have little influence on maternal behaviour since no improvements were noted in the diets prepared from the mothers' own food resources. In fact, there were indications of minor and unintended negative side effects as a result of the attention for the food ration: a slight tendency to stop breastfeeding at an earlier age, while the consumption of fresh milk was also found to be somewhat lower.

The younger that children are when they enrol in this kind of programme the better their nutritional status in the long run. Many children are from poor families where children generally show low weight levels and, in particular, incur relative weight losses after their first year of life. If children join the programme when this trend has already started the supplementation does only partly compensate for the sustained weight deficits. Children joining at an earlier age are less affected by these weight losses and tend to remain at their current growth level, and in terms of the programme objectives this can be considered a positive finding.

The fact that this result was achieved even though no changes in the utilization of own food resources were observed, indicates that the primary strength of this kind of intervention lies in the food supplementation rather than in the educational component. The present study does not address the important issue of possible sharing of food rations within the family, in particular sharing with siblings but also with adults. Until recently the tendency has been to regard such sharing as leakage. In the last few years, however, it has been suggested that it would be more appropriate and easier to look at food supplementation (or project food aid in general) as income transfer (Thomson, 1986). In this way any transfer of food to a family or individual is regarded as a resource transfer that can be given a certain value. This value can be measured and taken as the benefit, without distinguishing whether the food is eaten by a possible target child, eaten in addition to existing food resources, eaten instead of food that the family would otherwise have eaten, or even sold in the market. Although this line of reasoning has something of a disappearance trick, solving major problems of impact evaluation by a change of definitions, it does nevertheless point out an important area of future research (Katona-Apte, 1986).

Nutrition rehabilitation, the third type of intervention studied, usually faces an inherent dilemma, notably whether to concentrate on family education or whether to give the treatment of malnourished children priority. In the case of the Family Life Training Centres the policy has been to try to combine the two, although the programme does not comprise a medical component or medical back-up. In practice the centres also play a third role, namely that of temporary haven for mothers with domestic problems. In doing so, the programme clearly runs the risk of not being successful in either way. On the one hand educational facilities are meagre, on the other hand the nutritional regimen and medical supervision leave considerable room for improvement. The majority of children make satisfactory progress during their stay at the centres and in the six months afterwards. For most children this means that they gain weight at normal rates, although they do not show any catch-up growth. However, the weight gains of the youngest children were found to be rather small and a fair number of them did not show any weight increase at all at the centres. Furthermore, among the severely wasted children one in three did not show any weight recovery at the centre and nearly all the latter cases did not show satisfactory long-term progress either. It can be concluded that there is a need for close supervision of the feeding of children in nutrition rehabilitation centres, that the weight progress of children has to be carefully monitored, and that there is also need for close medical supervision for cases that do not show satisfactory progress during their stay at the centres.

Possible assistance after discharge from the centres is another important issue. Given the domestic circumstances of many women, notably their general lack of resources, the rehabilitation offered at the FLT centres does not offer a real solution to their problems. The centres are in a position to play a useful role in treating malnutrition among the first victims of poverty, young children, and can temporarily alleviate the difficult domestic situation of individual women.[1] Many cases potentially need long-term assistance. Because of the geographical distribution of cases, such assistance could best be provided through collaboration with other programmes that have a wider dispersion. This raises the general issue of co-operation between programmes. Existing collaboration usually did not go beyond incidental contacts between individual staff members, a number of PSH clinics organized at government health centres, and referral of malnourished cases from health centres to FLT centres. Generally, however, the three programmes operated separately, which is not surprising since two of them are the responsibility of different ministries and the third is run by a private organization. A serious shortcoming was the absence of an admission system by which cases could easily be referred from Health Centres to PSH clinics to FLT centres. Even more seriously lacking, perhaps, was a transferral system in the opposite direction, downwards so to speak, namely that cases discharged from FLT centres would be eligible for food supplementation at PSH clinics. At present these cases are not given priority for admission. In general the staff of nutrition rehabilitation centres are inclined to do the follow-up of cases themselves by means of home visits, but this is extremely time-consuming and requires transport facilities. In general it is not sufficiently realized that individual cases may belong to different target groups at different points in time. Consequently, it would be far more efficient if programmes could transfer cases to each other for follow-up.

In the final judgement it has to be admitted that the results of the three programmes are meagre at best. This does not mean that these programmes perform poorly compared with programmes elsewhere. Recent comprehensive reviews covering evaluations of nutrition programmes from various parts of the world also note the modest influence that interventions generally have, if impact is present at all. A review of food aid evaluations tells 'a rather dismal story and nutritional impact has rarely been substantiated' (Sahn, 1985: 2; Sahn & Pestronk, 1981). Other reviewers of child feeding programmes conclude that 'ongoing food distribution programmes seem to have relatively little impact' (Beaton, 1982: 1284; Beaton & Ghassemi, 1982). From a recent annotated bibliography on nutrition education in Third World countries it also appears that where impact was measured, it was usually found to be modest (Schurch & Wilquin, 1982). Although individual cases may occasionally show dramatic improvements after intervention, they stand beside many other cases that show less or no improvement at all.

Other experiences with rural development in developing countries have taught that it is generally unrealistic to expect spectacular improvements in economic conditions or wellbeing as a result of one particular intervention. Food and nutrition form an essential part of daily life and are closely interwoven with many other aspects of human existence and social organization, and these do not change overnight or even in a year's time. Moreover, and this must also be stressed, recipients usually represent only a small proportion of the total population, which inevitably reduces the social impact and importance of specific interventions. Really to change the nutritional situation of the target population would require a more comprehensive approach involving changes of a far wider nature than is attempted by the intervention programmes discussed in this monograph. This would mean a more sizeable and more consistent effort on the part of national governments, which would include not only better trained personnel and more financial resources, but also better organizational support and regular supervision of programmes. But, at the same time, it would also be necessary to find ways to improve the resource base of the families concerned and to pay more attention to individual children once they are in danger of becoming malnourished. Consequently, there should not be any overblown expectations of the impact of current interventions, and this in turn influences what can be demanded and expected of programme evaluation. A conclusion that can be drawn is that targeting of interventions is a sine qua non. In this way scarce resources can be better utilized and – which is perhaps equally important – the minor influence of interventions can be capitalized so that impact becomes more pronounced, thus measurable, subsequently researchable, and finally improvable.

8.3 Appraisal of Present Methodology

In view of the fact that the three programmes appear to produce little effect, a critical appraisal of the present evaluation methodology is required. Ultimately, there are two kinds of errors: false positive, concluding that effects exist where they do not exist; and false negative, concluding that no effects exist where they do indeed exist. In the former case, spurious differences may have been introduced by faulty selection of groups for comparison and it is this kind of error that usually receives most attention. In the latter case, either the study design or the selected indicators are not sufficiently sensitive to measure the perhaps minor effects of the respective interventions. The latter kind of error usually receives less attention, but it has been suggested that it is in fact the more common type of error and could be the reason for the reported absence of effects in many evaluation studies (Sahn, 1985).

The indicators used in the present studies were discussed in detail in Chapter 6; the same measuring instruments were satisfactorily used in the NIRP-survey and found to be discriminating. A number of findings of the programme evaluations further show that the indicators have sufficient discriminatory power. A case in point is the sensitization effect in respect of nutritional cognition demonstrated for the FLT-cases. Food consumption and anthropometry did reveal important differences between the programmes (and the control group), if not between conditions. The sensitivity of the designs is a more complex issue. The main point here is whether the conditions do in fact involve groups that differ sufficiently in contact with the programmes. Since different designs were used in the three studies, each is discussed in turn below.

The MCH study relies on a comparison between frequent and infrequent visitors to health centres. Theoretically, this comparison could be flawed if the first group consists of more motivated mothers who are more interested in providing good care for their children, in which case the comparison would reflect differences in motivation rather than effects of the intervention. We have tried to counter this possibility and there is good reason to believe that this was done with success. Although the aim of the study was to evaluate the Nutrition Field Workers, it turned out that their activities are organized in such a way that the research objective had to be formulated in more general terms, i.e. to establish the effects of the nutrition activities at MCH clinics with Field Workers. Although in this way no distinction is made between the influence of Nutrition Field Workers and other MCH workers, this seems acceptable because in practice their respective activities overlap considerably. Whatever the case, a possible error arising from this would be on the positive side and lead to false positive effects.

In the present case, however, there is a lack of positive impact and it is clearly not this kind of error that need concern us most, but rather whether the methodology was indeed sensitive enough to establish perhaps small effects. In other words the question is whether the two selected groups did indeed differ in their contact with the MCH services. Women were selected according to the frequency of contact with the health centres over the past few months, and their distance to the centres. Admittedly, the comparison is rather weak in the sense that groups might have been selected that differed more in their contact with the MCH services than the present groups. But in a general way the selection of the study groups accords with the way the Nutrition Field Workers operate: the evaluation as a reflection of the way the NFW programme operates in actual practice, not of what might be achieved under other more favourable circumstances.

The study has other limitations in that it does not assess nutritional improvements that are achieved over long periods of time. This applies in particular to any general diffusion of nutritional knowledge and nutritional effects of widespread immunization among the population at large.[2] None the less, the study as such is an attempt to evaluate the effects of nutrition instruction at health centres – a kind of intervention that is widespread in many developing countries.

The PSH evaluation consists of a comparison between recent and long-time participants. The latter group had participated in the programme for 33 months on average, a period quite long enough for the intervention to produce effects. The comparison rests on the assumption that the relevant characteristics of the mothers and children in the two respective groups were not different. However, examination of the weight records revealed that the children in the group of long-time participants, at the time of entry some years ago, were in much poorer condition than the children in the group of recent entrants. The analysis of nutritional status therefore concentrated on the development of the long-time participants over the years, without use of a comparison group.

The FLT evaluation used what is generally regarded as one of the more sensitive designs: pre-test–post-test. Women and children were examined at the start and shortly after the intervention as well as six months afterwards, and were compared with a control group examined twice over the same period of time. The control group differed from the FLT-cases in social–economic characteristics and in the nutritional status of children. On the one hand this gives a good insight into the background of the FLT-cases on the other hand it hampers the use of the control group. Among the FLT-cases there occurred a rate of attrition or about 25%: cases that could not be located at their homes afterwards. The rate in itself is not inordinately high, other researchers in similar circumstances encountered attrition rates of more than 50% (Gachuhi et al., 1972: 6). This means in effect that for this subgroup, the effects of the rehabilitation could not be assessed, but it does not detract from the evaluation of the remaining cases to which the study was consequently limited.

In evaluation, as in all research, there is a delicate balance between the false–positive and false–negative errors, outlined above. By evading the one, the other is invited. Given this inevitable dilemma and also given the limitations posed by the daily operations of the programmes, the three evaluations presented above each attempt to achieve an optimal balance between the extremes of lack of sensitivity and the introduction of spurious effects.

8.4 Evaluation[3]

The present volume is not intended as a manual on evaluation of nutrition intervention. For this we refer to Sahn et al. (1984), Schurch (1983) and an earlier textbook (Klein et al., 1979). The present monograph presents case studies of evaluation under the actual field conditions prevailing in developing countries. The essential features of evaluations under these conditions are three-fold. Firstly, there are the many methodological difficulties which almost invariably lead to imperfections of design, which either weaken the sensitivity of the evaluation, or alternatively restrict its scope. Secondly, the effects of most nutrition interventions in tropical countries are at best modest. Finally, nutrition programmes in tropical countries have to operate in an almost infinite variety of cultural settings, which not only raises practical implementation problems but which must inevitably have a strong bearing on the interpretation of evaluation findings as well.

The realization of this situation has elicited different reactions. Those concerned with the quality of the findings advocate stricter methodologies and more elaborate designs, while those concerned with the actual implementation of nutrition intervention stress the urgent need for further empirical insights, and often advocate a relaxation of methodological rigour. A practical suggestion in this connection is to look for so-called 'gross' outcomes in quick studies, before trying to establish 'net' outcomes with the help of stricter designs (Mason & Habicht, 1984). The danger, of course, is that the gross outcomes will start to lead a life of their own, and that the required further evaluation is not undertaken. The many and diverse cultural settings of nutrition programmes generally receive little attention, but they inevitably lead to a need for replication of programme evaluation under different conditions.

Sahn (1985) is inclined to attribute the general lack of effects to the insufficient sensitivity of most evaluations resulting from imperfections in indicators and, more often, from weaknesses in designs that mask any small effects. However, as described, design faults mostly take the form of the selection of groups that are spuriously different, i.e. groups that will show themselves to be different on outcome measures for the wrong reasons. This type of error would therefore result in a greater number of significant findings (albeit unwarranted). But this is not the case and it is unlikely that researchers have leant over backwards, as it were, making errors in the opposite direction by selecting groups that are not sufficiently different in exposure.

The studies that do report effects are often discredited as having methodological weaknesses and leaving room for possible alternative explanations. As argued earlier, this is inherent to the very nature of non-experimental methods. The problem is not so much that imperfections exist, but how to cope with them. The intelligent use of findings from different studies can lead to an overall picture which is more convincing than any one particular set of data. And, in this sense, evaluation is no different from social research in general, where only the existence of mutually supporting but independent data sets eventually leads to accepted theoretical insights.

There is a finer point of methodology that needs mentioning. Experimental (and quasi-experimental) research is based on a model of scientific inquiry, in which it is up to the researcher to prove that differences exist between naturally different or experimentally created conditions. In the absence of such proof it is assumed that there are no differences which, however, is not the same as proof that *no* differences exist. In fact, usually there is a gamut of differences which are not statistically significant, but which can either reflect chance variations or which may reflect – and in a number of cases must reflect – genuine, but small, effects.

Instead, there is a strong tendency to strive for a 'crucial' evaluation, in analogy of the 'crucial experiment', the mythical study that will give a final answer once and for all. And in this case the answer is usually wanted quickly as well. In the case of nutrition interventions in Third World countries, this research approach is not realistic. Not only are there many different types of programmes, but similar programmes have to work among very different population groups and often under unique circumstances. In Kenya, for example, there are between thirty and forty ethnic groups that differ in child-rearing habits and dietary practices. Each nutrition programme therefore faces a multitude of conducive or hindering conditions which means that there is no single 'best' intervention, but that certain interventions function more effectively under certain conditions, and it is on this aspect that attention should focus. Evaluation should not be conceptualized as providing a set of ultimate and objective standards for sudden-death decisions to continue or terminate a particular programme. Nutrition programmes generally exist because there is a 'felt need', either humanitarian or political, and the contribution of evaluation is more in the nature of helping to seek the optimal combination of local conditions and type of assistance offered.

Evaluations must therefore be prepared to assess very different interventions and to look for small differences against a background of profound social–economic variations. This suggests several possible research strategies. One is improved control over study conditions; other alternatives being to pay more attention to the analysis of 'weak' statistical effects and to use other than quantitative research methods. The analysis of so-called weak statistical effects requires series of similar studies of similar programmes to be undertaken; the studies in this monograph form an example of this approach. Qualitative research methods, notably of an anthropological nature, provide behavioural insights which may eventually suggest programme improvements, but which generally do not give a straightforward answer as to whether the intervention has an effect or not. Usually, however, a solution to the evaluation dilemma is sought in improved study designs with greater control over non-treatment variables. This is not only difficult to realize, it is nearly always costly and time-consuming. These measures, however, are firstly aimed at measuring the final impact of nutrition programmes.

A comprehensive bibliography concludes that there is a general agreement among authors that evaluation should be a routine programme activity, that field staff must be involved at all stages and that any results should rapidly be fed into the programme concerned (Burgess, 1982). It is in this perspective that the calls for so-called 'in-built monitoring and evaluation' must be seen. These monitoring and evaluation ('m&e') systems are, in principle, designed to monitor the flow of project inputs and outputs and to evaluate not only the effects of intervention in a restricted way but also the impact in a wider sense (Miller & Sahn, 1984). 'M&e' systems usually have two lofty and laudable objectives: to place more emphasis on the need for systematic monitoring and routine process evaluation, and to keep the total costs of monitoring and evaluation low. However, they are too often depicted as a kind of 'miracle' package of process evaluation and impact evaluation, together with involvement of local personnel which, on top of all this, would be low in costs as well (Gotzman, 1986).

The proposed 'm&e' systems have severe limitations as regards the topics that can be covered and subsequent insights that can be gained, but they also face severe restrictions as regards the type and reliability of data that can be collected, and the availability, accuracy and motivation of project staff. The few examples of such systems functioning in actual practice show that they exist only by the grace of qualified research personnel, as in the Philippines, or thanks to the involvement of local research consultants, as in Bangladesh, and that they are nevertheless quite restricted in scope (Munger, 1983; Hartog & Leemhuis, 1985).

The question must be raised, however, whether impact evaluation does not often receive undue emphasis, to the detriment of process evaluation. One must seriously doubt the need and feasibility for in-built, that is continuous, evaluation of impact among recipients if the impact is of such elusive nature as behavioural changes among mothers and developmental improvement of children. Process evaluation on the other hand is also necessary, notably on a day-to-day basis, to assure the proper delivery of services. In principle, the necessary monitoring can be done routinely by permanent project staff, at the same time providing an essential data source on which to graft later impact evaluation.

Nevertheless, there are profound differences in the aims, execution and requirements between the two kinds of evaluation. Impact evaluation requires data to be aggregated and compared across carefully selected subgroups, while as often as not data on non-participants are needed as well for purposes of comparison. Moreover, information is often needed that cannot be collected routinely by project staff, either because they lack the necessary training or simply because they lack the time. There is no doubt that 'm&e' systems require so-called extra or special studies which either address typical impact issues or which test behavioural assumptions underlying the intervention as such (Sahn, 1985). In fact, it may be more useful to speak of different stages in the evaluation of ongoing programmes (Mason & Habicht, 1984).

Ultimately the aim of monitoring and evaluation is to gain information about the daily functioning of nutrition intervention programmes and about their effects. The quality of such information and possible ensuing insights are determined by the issues that are addressed. The more fundamental these issues are the higher the costs of research. In this sense, it is inevitable that as soon as monitoring and evaluation systems are genuinely directed at impact evaluation, they run into the same problems that others have come to experience. Where exactly process evaluation ends and impact evaluation begins is not always clear, but in its final form impact evaluation is concerned with behavioural research, and this is expensive, requires expert personnel and takes time. Firstly, there are the many methodological difficulties that bedevil evaluation of programmes in general, but particularly programmes already operating under field conditions. The programmes, moreover, not only differ among one another, they also have to operate in many different cultural settings. The impact of most interventions furthermore is small, be it cognitional, behavioural or nutritional and this makes improvements difficult to quantify. Evaluations, like the actual interventions, have to operate under limiting conditions which restrict their potential contributions, and that certainly does not make them the definitive arbiters that they are often expected to be. Evaluation is a tool, a tool that has to be used carefully and skilfully and as such is an important, but modest, means to achieve improvements and to realize the necessary targeting. Riecken (1979) has remarked that one can only expect the quality of evaluation for which one is prepared to pay, financially but also in terms of effort and interference with daily operations. Programme managers, officials and politicians must weigh the costs against the possible insights that can be gained. Ultimately, the costs and benefits of evaluation itself have to be weighed against each other.

Appendix 1
NIRP-Survey: Food Consumption of Pre-School Children[1]

1A
Children consuming foods listed (%)

	Breast-fed	1yr	2yr	3–4yr	Total (N=300)
Cereals					
maize, fresh	07	01	07	04	04.6
maize, dry	02	15	20	50	22.3
maize, flour	37	38	53	66	49.4
maize, flour, brand	37	21	15	12	18.4
maize-soya, flour	—	—	—	—	00.2
finger millet, flour	—	—	—	—	01.6
rice	02	05	05	03	04.4
sorghum, flour	09	13	17	04	12.2
wheat, flour	04	03	07	04	05.1
Roots, tubers & starchy fruits					
banana	57	62	40	39	48.0
potato, Irish	33	40	29	28	32.6

1B
Average amount of food consumed (g)

	Total (N=300)	Breast-fed	1yr	2yr	3–4yr
Cereals					
maize, fresh	04.0	03	01	05	06
maize, dry	21.9	01	11	24	46
maize, flour	42.2	24	30	51	53
maize, flour, brand	15.1	23	22	12	08
maize-soya, flour	00.1	—	—	—	—
finger millet, flour	00.3	—	—	—	—
rice	02.7	04	02	03	03
sorghum, flour	05.1	04	06	07	02
wheat, flour	05.1	03	03	06	08
Total	96.5	62	75	108	126
Roots, tubers & starchy fruits					
banana	86.5	117	123	69	50
potato, Irish	30.8	35	43	25	22

1A
Children consuming foods listed (%)

	Breast-fed	1yr	2yr	3–4yr	Total (N=300)
potato, sweet	09	16	19	13	15.5
taro	02	12	05	10	08.1
Total					
Grain legumes					
beans, kidney; dry	33	37	60	63	50.6
peas, pigeon; dry	—	—	—	—	01.2
beans, peas; fresh	—	—	—	—	00.9
Total					
Vegetables					
carrots	—	—	—	—	01.4
eggplant/squash	—	—	—	—	02.3
leaves, light green	09	08	08	13	09.0
leaves, medium green	—	—	—	—	00.5
leaves, dark green	17	25	29	36	28.1

1B
Average amount of food consumed (g)

	Total (N=300)	Breast-fed	1yr	2yr	3–4yr
potato, sweet	51.4	32	42	72	35
taro	15.6	03	20	10	26
Total	184.3	187	228	176	133
Grain legumes					
beans, kidney; dry	51.4	35	41	67	44
peas, pigeon; dry	00.5	—	—	—	—
beans, peas; fresh	01.7	—	—	—	—
Total	53.6	35	41	67	44
Vegetables					
carrots	00.6	—	—	—	—
eggplant/squash	02.0	—	—	—	—
leaves, light green	08.6	08	05	09	13
leaves, medium green	00.9	—	—	—	—
leaves, dark green	28.5	24	24	29	36

02	02	07	10	05.8	pumpkin	08.0	06	01	09	17
07	12	06	11	08.8	tomato	01.0	01	02	—	01
					Total	49.6	39	32	47	67
					Fruits					
—	—	—	—	00.7	avocado pear	01.8	—	—	—	—
—	—	—	—	01.4	lemon	00.3	—	—	—	—
—	—	—	—	01.8	mango	02.6	—	—	—	—
—	—	—	—	01.2	orange/tangerine	02.1	—	—	—	—
—	—	—	—	01.6	passion fruit	00.8	—	—	—	—
—	—	—	—	00.2	paw paw	00.2	—	—	—	—
—	—	—	—	00.2	pineapple	00.3	—	—	—	—
—	—	—	—	00.2	plums	00.8	—	—	—	—
					Total	08.9	—	—	—	—
					Meats & animal products					
—	—	—	—	00.5	chicken	00.1	—	—	—	—
09	18	08	06	10.6	egg	04.7	02	10	03	03
—	—	—	—	03.2	meat (beef, goat)	01.5	—	—	—	—
89	95	87	91	90.7	milk, fresh	319.6	278	435	276	255
—	—	—	—	00.5	milkpowder, skimmed	00.1	—	—	—	—

1A

Children consuming foods listed (%)

	Breast-fed	1yr	2yr	3–4yr	Total (N=300)
milk, sour	—	—	—	—	00.5
milk, goat	—	—	—	—	00.2
liver	—	—	—	—	00.2
Total					
Miscellaneous					
bread	07	10	07	13	09.2
cacao	—	—	—	—	00.9
cacao drink	—	—	—	—	00.7
fat	63	70	73	71	70.5
sugar	70	71	82	81	77.1
sugar cane	—	—	—	—	00.9
soft drinks, syrup	—	—	—	—	00.2

Breast-fed Age Group[2]

1B

Average amount of food consumed (g)

	Total (N=300)	Breast-fed	1yr	2yr	3–4yr
milk, sour	00.9	—	—	—	—
milk, goat	00.9	—	—	—	—
liver	00.1	—	—	—	—
Total	327.9	280	445	279	258
Miscellaneous					
bread	07.8	03	09	05	15
cacao	00.1	—	—	—	—
cacao drink	00.02	—	04	—	—
fat	03.8	04	04	04	04
sugar	18.5	13	18	20	19
sugar cane	00.6	—	—	—	—
soft drinks, syrup	00.2	—	—	—	—
Total	31.0	20	31	29	38

Breast-fed Age Group

[1] No breakdown by age group is given for foods that were consumed by less than 10 children (or 3.3% of all cases).
[2] BF (N=31); 1yr (N=87); 2yr (N=113); 3–4yr (N=57).
An explanation of the uneven distribution of cases is given in Chapter 4, note 4.
Source: HNS, 1984

Appendix 2
NIRP-Survey: Weight and Height of Pre-School Children
by Half-Yearly Age Groups (Children, 6–59 months)

Age (months)	Weight (kg)					
	N^1	Boys average	s.d.	N	Girls average	s.d.
06–11	31	07.8	1.1	33	07.3	1.7
12–17	50	09.2	1.2	26	08.6	0.8
18–23	42	10.1	1.2	45	09.9	1.1
24–29	36	10.9	1.5	60	10.8	1.4
30–35	38	11.9	1.4	47	11.6	1.4
36–41	41	12.9	1.7	47	12.7	1.4
42–47	45	13.9	1.3	28	13.9	1.4
48–53	50	14.6	1.7	34	14.4	1.3
54–59	51	15.4	1.3	39	14.2	1.6

Age (months)	Height (cm)					
	N^1	Boys average	s.d.	N	Girls average	s.d.
06–11	31	67.6	3.0	33	66.7	4.2
12–17	50	73.4	2.5	26	73.0	2.5
18–23	42	78.4	3.7	45	77.6	3.5
24–29	36	83.1	4.7	60	81.2	4.5
30–35	38	87.7	4.0	47	86.9	4.0
36–41	41	91.0	5.9	47	91.4	4.1
42–47	45	94.5	4.2	28	94.9	5.6
48–53	50	97.9	5.7	34	98.1	4.1
54–59	51	101.7	3.7	39	98.1	4.9

[1] Weighted numbers (raw total: 265 boys; 242 girls)
Source: HNS, 1983: 85, 91

Appendix 3
NIRP-Survey: Anthropometric Indices of Pre-School Children by Three-Monthly Age Groups (Children, 6–59 months)

Age (months)	N^1	Average height for age	Average weight for height	Average weight for age	Percent children below critical value of H-A (90)	W-H (90)	W-A (80)
6–8	29	97.2	96.4	90.0	0.0	31.0	20.7
9–11	35	95.0	96.8	86.3	11.4	25.7	25.7
12–14	37	95.3	95.3	87.3	0.0	24.3	21.6
15–17	39	92.9	94.8	84.7	20.5	30.8	41.0
18–20	40	93.7	93.3	84.6	20.0	35.0	35.0
21–23	47	92.0	96.0	85.4	31.9	17.0	27.7
24–26	55	92.1	96.4	86.0	29.1	18.2	25.5
27–29	41	92.2	95.1	84.9	34.1	26.8	29.3
30–32	43	93.1	96.0	86.3	25.6	18.6	23.3
33–35	42	93.5	92.2	83.0	14.3	45.2	31.0
36–38	37	92.2	94.2	83.1	29.7	24.3	37.8
39–41	51	94.1	96.4	87.4	21.6	17.6	27.5
42–44	38	93.9	96.7	87.3	18.4	13.2	26.3
45–47	35	93.3	98.9	87.9	31.4	2.9	8.6
48–50	34	94.1	97.5	87.7	8.8	11.8	23.5
51–53	50	92.9	95.7	84.7	22.0	20.0	32.0
54–56	39	92.3	94.7	82.7	17.9	15.4	33.3
57–59	51	93.0	95.6	84.1	23.5	23.5	31.4
Total	743	93.4	95.6	85.6	20.9	22.2	28.1
(s.d.)		(4.5)	(7.9)	(10.3)			

^{1} Weighted numbers (Raw total = 509)

Appendix 4
Review of Evaluation Studies and Characteristics of the Respondents

	Nutrition Field Workers		Pre-School Health Progr.		Family Life Training Centres			Control Group	
	Infreq. visitors	Frequent visitors	Recent particip.	Long-time particip.	Admission	Discharge	Home visit	1st exam.	2nd exam.
Period of study (1978)	Nov–Dec		March–April		March–June		Oct.	March–May	Oct–Nov
Number of cases									
Zone 2	24	25	23	25	19	id.	id.	—	—
Borderline 2/3	—	—	—	—	—	—	—	50	id.
Zone 3	32	40	25	32	19	id.	id.	—	—
Borderline 3/4	—	—	—	—	—	—	—	50	id.
Zone 4	27	26	22	25	23	id.	id.	—	—
Total	83	91	70	82	61	id.	id.	100	id.
Type of data collected									
Nutr. knowledge	partial	partial	vv	vv	vv	vv	vv	vv	vv
Nutr. preferences	vv	vv	vv	vv	vv	vv	vv	vv	vv
Dietary recall	vv	vv	vv	vv	=	=	vv	vv	vv
Anthropometry	vv	vv	vv	vv	vv	vv	vv	vv	vv
Size (average)	5.6	6.4	6.5	6.7	6.9	id.	id.	6.9	id.
Characteristics: Households (%)									
Income group									
poor	61[1]	63[1]	39	55	66	id.	id.	42	id.
medium	33[1]	28[1]	50	39	30	id.	id.	35	id.
rich	06[1]	10[1]	11	06	05	id.	id.	23	id.

Characteristics: Mother (%)	Nutrition Field Workers		Pre-School Health Progr.		Family Life Training Centres			Control Group	
	Infreq. visitors	Frequent visitors	Recent particip.	Long-time particip.	Admission	Discharge	Home visit	1st exam.	2nd exam.
Domestic stage									
young	46	37	30	23	20	id.	id.	24	id.
middle-stage	42	51	61	63	69	id.	id.	55	id.
senior	12	12	09	13	12	id.	id.	21	id.
No. pre-school children									
few (1–2)	67	67	61	70	52	id.	id.	65	id.
several (3 or more)	33	33	39	30	48	id.	id.	35	id.
Farm size (acres)									
no land	22	25	03	07	42	id.	id.	00	id.
0.1–0.9	11	11	31	33	12	id.	id.	31	id.
1.0–2.9	38	35	26	28	17	id.	id.	52	id.
3.0 or more	30	29	40	31	29	id.	id.	16	id.
Age									
19 yrs and younger	13	09	03	—	02	id.	id.	05	id.
20–29 yrs	59	57	53	44	44	id.	id.	36	id.
30–49 yrs	25	34	41	56	53	id.	id.	57	id.
50 yrs and over	02	—	03	—	02	id.	id.	02	id.
Education									
none	39	35	40	49	54	id.	id.	34	id.
standard 1–4	19	15	17	26	25	id.	id.	34	id.

144

Characteristics: Children (%)

standard 5–7(8)	39	43	37	24	16	id.	id.	25
secondary	04	07	06	01	—	id.	id.	08
Marital status								
single	12	17	04	04	10	id.	id.	01
married, monogam.	86	76	86	85	61	id.	id.	90
married, polygam.	n.a.		04	04	10	id.	id.	02
separated/divorced	01	06	04	05	16	id.	id.	02
widowed	01	02	01	02	03	id.	id.	05
Age distribution of children for whom dietary recall was recorded								
Breastfed (BF)	27	26	28	08	—	14	id.	15
06–23 months (1 yr)	31	35	25	12	—	20	id.	17
24–35 months (2 yr)	11	18	12	15	—	22	id.	31
36–59 months (3–4 yr)	14	12	03	41	—	05	id.	29
Total	83	91	68	76	—	61	id.	92
Age distribution of children for whom anthropometry was recorded								
06–11 months	26	27	18	00	18	id.	id.	11
12–23 months	32	34	39	03	24	id.	id.	33
24–35 months	11	18	19	08	21	id.	id.	33
36–59 months	14	12	17	77	31	id.	id.	69
Total	83	91	93	88	94	id.	id.	146

[1] Percentages not comparable with figures for the other programmes. See Chapter 6, note 6 (p. 153).

145

Notes

Chapter 1

[1] At present, this approach is being extended to include the evaluation of the nutritional effects of rural development programmes (Niemeijer et al., 1985; 1988; FNSP, 1985).
[2] A comprehensive bibliography on nutrition in Kenya by Jansen et al. (1987) has recently been published.
[3] The differences in sample composition mainly concern differences in age range. The three CBS-surveys do not cover the northern part of the country, thus excluding about 5% of the population.

Chapter 2

[1] Other outcomes, for example increased energy expenditure or improved cognitive development, are remote or very difficult to measure and can hardly serve as indicators.
[2] All female guardians of children and all women bringing children to the programmes are referred to as 'mothers'. Very few children do not live with their parents and fewer than 5% of the children were brought to the programmes by someone other than their mother.
[3] Sampling was based on the holdings in the areas as registered at the land office. The survey concentrated on children in the age range of 6–59 months and holdings where there was at least one household with children in that age range were selected for study. Holdings where no people resided and holdings occupied by households without young children were excluded. From each holding one household with child(ren) in this age range was selected, except when four or more such households were present (5% of the cases), in which case more than

one was selected. The 300 households visited represented a total of 439 eligible households resident on 284 holdings. Since certain households represent other households (on the same holding) that were not visited, all data were weighted accordingly to obtain estimates for the total population (HNS, 1983, 1984).

[4] Kiiriangoro lies at an altitude of approximately 1650m, Kagurumo at an altitude of between 1400m and 1450m. Estimated rainfall per year is 1600mm and 1100mm respectively (Jaetzold & Schmidt, 1983: 569).

[5] Rainfall at Kiambu station in 1977 and 1978 was 1464mm and 1473mm respectively, compared with an average of 1073mm for that station during the period 1975–82. Rainfall at the other end of the province, in Nyeri, was 905mm and 1018mm respectively, with an average figure of 931mm between 1975 and 1982 (CBS, 1983a). Official estimates of maize production in Central Province during these two years were 1.62 and 1.87 million bags, compared with an annual average of 1.91 million bags over the period 1976–81 (CBS, 1976–81).

Chapter 3

[1] Ecological zones V (arid) and VI (very arid) do not exist in Central Province. Zone I, moorland, grassland and barren land at high altitudes, does occur but is largely uninhabited and of no relevance to this research.

[2] These densities were calculated for the administrative locations in which the respective programmes are situated (MoFEP, 1970). For the Limuru research area this relates to the Lari and Limuru locations; for the Kandara area the Muruka, Gaichanjiru and Kigumo locations; and for the Mwea area the locations of Tebere, Murinduko and Mutithi. During the 1979 census the boundaries of Lari location were redrawn and the location was considerably enlarged with less densely populated land situated on the escarpment. The figures presented in the text have been adjusted in this respect wherever possible. They were calculated on the basis of the sub-locations included in the 1969 census, although the boundaries of several of these sub-locations had also been redrawn, and Kijabe sub-location had to be excluded from the calculation for that reason.

[3] Between 1974 and 1978 the Central Bureau of Statistics carried out a series of household surveys, called the Integrated Rural Surveys (CBS, 1981a). The fourth survey in 1978 gives the most relevant information for our purposes, and is referred to as IRS-4.

[4] At the time of land consolidation in Central Province, three acres was generally regarded as the minimum 'economic' farm size (Sorrenson, 1967).

[5] In the two ecological zones in Kigumo Division, covered in the NIRP-survey, the percentage of households cultivating food crops was as follows (N=300):

Intervention in Child Nutrition (Kenya)

	Upper location (Kiiriangoro)	Lower location (Kagurumo)
Maize	97	100
Beans	94	100
Peas	5	27
Bananas	95	82
Roots & tubers	82	91
Vegetables	67	69
Fruits	35	56
Seasonings	21	16

Source: HNS, 1983: 32

[6] The Integrated Rural Survey survey includes a high percentage of 'not stated' cases (17%).

[7] As a consequence of the prevailing high coffee prices, coffee offered the best opportunities in terms of gross cash returns. It was estimated that in 1977, horticultural crops fetched 2000KSh/acre on average, rice 1560KSh/acre and coffee 15,700KSh/acre, but this last figure should be seen in perspective. Few farmers grow more than half an acre of coffee, and because cultivation methods are often less than optimal their harvests are usually modest. It was calculated that in the top year, 1977, some 85% of the coffee-growing smallholders in Murang'a earned an average total of only 4000KSh from this crop (Meilink, 1979: 22, 28).

[8] Reported percentages of the population over 15 years working regularly on selected crops are as follows:

	Maize			Coffee		
	P	W	H	P	W	H
Females	91	91	91	31	35	32
Males	37	42	42	21	22	20

P = Planting; W = Weeding; H = Harvesting
Source: CBS, 1981a: 74, 76

[9] Day-labour should not be confused with communal labour, the traditional help given to neighbours, for example when building a house. This kind of assistance, however, appears to be on the decline.

[10] The different studies listed in Table 3 aim to assess the actual incidence of poverty in the rural areas. The division into income groups used here and in the NIRP-survey serves for purposes of analysis, and as such was not meant to quantify the absolute incidence of rural poverty in Central Province.

[11] By Kenyan standards, the divorce rate among the Kikuyu is average. A recent national survey found that among Kikuyu women who had first married during the past ten years, the marriage had been dissolved in 11% of the cases. Among the national population this figure was also 11%, while rates for different ethnic groups ranged from 3% (Kalenjin) to 20% (Kambaa) and 22% (Mijikenda) (CBS, 1980: 79).

148

[12] Two or more minor activities, i.e. if foods crops were sold occasionally, and/or 0.3 acre was planted with coffee, and/or 4 cows were owned, and/or 10 chickens were kept.

[13] According to NIRP-survey, 33% of the households in Kigumo Division were classified as commercial farmers. In order, the following percentages of households met the respective qualifications:

(a)	0.5 acre under cash crop	16.9
(b)	regular sale of food crops	0.5
(c)	two minor activities	8.9
(d)	employ farm labour	7.1

[14] In Kigumo Division the distribution of off-farm employment among husbands (household heads), already mentioned on page 36, was as follows:

(a)	employment with government/industry	35	
(b)	self-employed	17	
	Regular Employment		52
(c)	casual labour	35	
(d)	no off-farm employment	13	
	No Regular Employment		48

[15] Combined distribution of commercial farming and off-farm employment is as follows:

Income group	Employment	Farming	%
Rich households	Regular	Commercial	21
{Medium households}	Regular	Not commercial	26
{Medium households}	Not regular	Commercial	12
Poor households	Not regular	Not commercial	41

Source: HNS, 1983: 44 (N=300)

[16] The type of roof, thatched or corrugated iron, has often been used to indicate differences in wealth. By now, however, thatch is becoming a rare commodity in most of Central Province and a thatched roof is at least as expensive as one of corrugated iron.

[17] The definition of 'young' families is households in which all children are still under six, i.e. 72 months of age. This age limit should not be confused with the age of 59 months, marking the limit of the main subject of the present studies, the pre-school children.

[18] As cross-tabulation of households in the NIRP-survey shows:

Income group	Domestic stage			Total (%)
	Young (%)	Middle (%)	Senior (%)	
Poor	25	60	16	100
Medium	24	54	21	100
Rich	22	66	12	100

Source: HNS, 1983: 50, 52 (N=300)

[19] As also shown by cross-tabulation of households in the NIRP-survey:

Income group	No. of pre-school children		
	1–2 (%)	3+ (%)	Total (%)
Poor	69	31	100
Medium	64	36	100
Rich	63	37	100

Source: HNS, 1983: 50, 52 (N=300)

[20] Again as shown from cross-tabulation of the NIRP households, although in this case the relation is not fully independent. Among the young families, the percentage of families with three or more pre-school children is understandably smaller because of the presence of young couples that have recently married. The same applies to the senior families because this latter category also covers women nearing the end of their reproductive cycle:

Domestic stage	No. of pre-school children		
	1–2 (%)	3+ (%)	Total (%)
Young	79	21	100
Middle	58	42	100
Senior	70	30	100

Source: HNS, 1983: 50, 52 (N=300)

Chapter 4

1 Where reference is made in the text to beans, bananas, or potatoes without further specification, kidney beans, green (cooking) bananas and Irish potatoes are meant.

[2] For reasons of convenience we will, from here on, refer to the group of roots, tubers and starchy fruits as 'roots & tubers' in short, and which therefore also includes green bananas.

[3] With the exception of Rift Valley Province where the frequency of milk consumption is also high, although lower than in Central Province, and with the possible exception of pastoralist populations, on which few data exist.

[4] Food consumption data were collected by means of the 24-hour recall method. In survey households with more than one child, aged 6–59 months, the recall was recorded for the child nearest to two years of age. The method makes no allowance for the consumption of breastmilk and, consequently, the reported food intake of breastfed children is incomplete.

[5] It is possible that milk availability shows seasonal variations as a result

of differences in feeding animals at different times of the year. If such variation were in turn to result in variations in the milk consumption of young children, the time of the survey would not show peak consumption, since it coincides with the end of the dry season and the beginning of the rains.

[6] CBS (1979a) reports that 30% of the children's porridge prepared still includes millet, which suggests a higher rate of consumption than the NIRP findings indicate.

[7] All children still being breastfed are included in the group BF, irrespective of age. The group includes only two children over 24 months and the average age of the children in this group is lower than that of the next group, which comprises the children between 6–23 months who are no longer breastfed.

[8] This region includes not only Central Province but also adjoining Eastern Province.

[9] The children included in the NFW study; see Chapter 6.1, p. 92.

[10] The technique used in this analysis (a purely statistical search for subgroups with nutritional problems) often leads to results which are difficult to interpret, such as the finding that 'ownership of a holding' is a condition contributing to childhood malnutrition.

Chapter 5

[1] To give an example of how attendance is organized: at Gaichanjiru Mission Hospital a PSH clinic was held three mornings a week, that is twelve clinics a month which, with an average attendance of about 40 children, amounts to a total enrolment of 500 children.

[2] On average a mother has to wait some 25 minutes for her child to be weighed. The weighing takes, on average, no more than two minutes, and this includes the individual advice given to mothers whose children show little or no progress. After that she has to wait about 45–50 minutes for the beginning of the lecture, which usually takes 20 minutes. After that she generally has to wait another 20 minutes before it is her turn to receive foods. (Observations on five occasions at the three centres concerned; time records for 229 mothers) (HN, 1980b: 22).

[3] The authorized food rations, at the time, consisted of 1.0kg of oil, 2.0kg of bulgar wheat and 2.0kg of corn–soya mixture (the latter sometimes replaced by dried skimmed milk). The actual rations issued, however, have been estimated to reach only 75% of the authorized amounts, on average (PCI, 1980). The energy provided by the latter amount is about 17,000kcal. and 500g protein. This is 575kcal./day, which is about 30% of the energy requirements of young children in the age groups concerned.

[4] In the course of 1977/78, the period of the present studies, the potential PSH beneficiaries were redefined, so as to include the mothers of the

children. This meant that mothers could receive an extra food ration for their own consumption; otherwise the clinics continued to function as usual.

[5] The total number of cottages/rooms at the three centres is 32, and the average period of residence is about three weeks. If the centres are open eleven months a year, and only one mother is accommodated per cottage (although more is possible), 384 women could be admitted per year.

[6] As regards the number of potential cases: the total population of the three districts was estimated to be 1,500,000 in 1978 (CBS, 1972: 3), of which 10–11% were children between the ages of 12 and 48 months, or 150,000 children. According to the CBS nutrition surveys and the NIRP-survey, 1% of the children in this age range are below W-A(60) and are severely malnourished. This means 1500 children at any one time; the total number per year should be higher. During 1978 the total number of children admitted in such severe condition was less than 135 (HN, 1979: 6, 24, 30). Even assuming that the FLT centres serve only the divisions in which they are situated, the rate of admissions could be higher. (Total estimated population of Limuru, Kigumo and Mwea divisions: 302,000; children aged 12–48 months: 30,000; estimated number of children with W-A $<$ 60, at any one time: 300; more over the whole year.)

[7] The figures listed in Table 13 are drawn from different sources; for the survey population (HNS, 1983) and for the FLT programme, the cases introduced in Chapter 4.6 (HN, 1982). The characteristics listed for the PSH programme are those for the combined groups of recent and long-time participants as described in Chapter 6.1 (HN, 1980b). The characteristics of the MCH population presented have not been reported before and were collected during a preliminary survey of the general characteristics of MCH visitors at the three selected health centres.

[8] Further analysis showed that in Gaichanjiru, the PSH clinic nearest and most similar to the NIRP-survey areas, over 70% of the PSH participants came from households classified as poor (HN, 1980b: 40).

Chapter 6

[1] See Chapter 2, note 1.

[2] The selection criteria at Kandara health centre are slightly different. Frequent visitors were defined as women who had to travel for an hour or less and who had attended five times or more during the previous six months. Infrequent visitors were women who had to travel for more than an hour and who had attended four times or less over the previous six months.

The difference in selection criteria between the centres came about because the above requirements had been formulated on the basis of observations in Kandara, the first centre studied. It turned out, however, that with these criteria the number of available subjects at the two other centres was drastically reduced. The criteria in Lari and Kimbimbi were therefore slightly modified and they are the ones listed in the main text.

³ Not included were women who reported that they usually attended at another health facility because this posed an unacceptable interference with the design. Also excluded from the study were the very few non-Kikuyu and the very few men who brought their children to the MCH clinics.

⁴ The survey households were seen again after another period of six months during a third visit.

⁵ It must be pointed out, however, that the different groups were not all examined at the same time of the year, so that the possibility of seasonal differences exists.

⁶ By force of circumstance there was less time available for individual interviews at the health centres than at the PSH clinics and FLT centres. This meant that a shortened socio-economic questionnaire had to be used. The stratification in the MCH study is therefore based on an approximation.

There is reasonable agreement between the resulting division and the final division into income groups used in the NIRP-survey (Gamma = .60) and in the two other evaluation studies (HN, 1980a: 46–7). However, it must be pointed out that the distribution of income groups in the MCH study cannot be compared directly with that in the other studies and this can explain why more households in the MCH study were classified as belonging to the 'poor' income group.

⁷ The four supplementary foods inquired after were: ucuru; gitoero; beans; and maize meal with vegetables.

⁸ The 16 comparisons included in the schedule are the following:
(−) beans–rice, (−) beans–finger millet, (−) beans–green banana, (−) beans–cabbage;
(−) peas–maize flour, (−) peas–kale, (−) peas–Irish potato, (−) peas–orange;
(−) eggs–rice, (−) eggs–finger millet, (−) eggs–green banana, (−) eggs–cabbage;
(−) meat–maize flour, (−) meat–kale, (−) meat–Irish potato, (−) meat–orange.

The actual interviews that were employed included a further eight comparisons between cereals, roots & tubers, vegetables and fruits. These additional items were included in the presentation of NIRP-survey results (HNS, 1984), but were not included in the analysis of the evaluation studies.

⁹ Design copied by courtesy of the Central Bureau of Statistics.

¹⁰ Among the FLT-cases no inquiries were made after food consumption at admission and discharge. At discharge interviews would have reflected the diets at the centres, and at admission the same would usually have been the case because mothers were not necessarily interviewed on the very first day at the centre. Even if mothers had been interviewed on that day, many of the children were at that time in serious condition and their food consumption consequently affected. Furthermore it must be noted that the heights of FLT-children were not measured at discharge, because significant changes in height were not expected after the short stay at the centre.

Among the control group nutritional knowledge was not examined during the revisit because no good reasons could be given to the respondents for this repeated inquiry. Furthermore, height was not recorded during the first revisit to the control group because the senior staff who measured length were not able to visit households personally at that time. Heights were, however, measured during a third visit after one year, so that growth rates over the period of study can still be calculated.

Chapter 7

[1] $F = 4.22$; $p < 05$.

[2] A similar trend was observed among MCH-visitors; in this case, however, around the division line of 21 months. Among the infrequent visitors, 38% of the women preferred to breastfeed for longer than 21 months; among the frequent visitors this was 23%.

[3] The difference in preference score among the two FLT examinations is the result of repeated interviewing, as the similar increase in scores among the control group indicates (HN, 1982: 37).

[4] $t = 2.24$; $p < 05$.

[5] This was mainly caused by the PSH-participants. The long-time participants having been admitted some 2.5 years ago, these children are generally older than the recent participants. For that reason, age overlap between the two study conditions was deliberately created by including the younger siblings of the long-time participants in the study as well and by recording the food intake of the child nearest to two years of age in the household, and restricting the comparison to children in the age range of 6–35 months.

[6] See Chapter 6, note 10.

[7] At first sight the poorer condition of this group at admission could be attributed to the larger percentage of participants stemming from poor households. Detailed analysis, however, showed that this is not the case (HN, 1980b: 42).

[8] The weights recorded by the clinic staff proved sufficiently accurate. Weights taken by the NIRP team at the time of the study corresponded closely with those recorded by clinic staff on the same occasion ($r=.91$).

[9] All children of the 61 mothers in the study were included in the analysis. An alternative would have been to include only one child per mother in the analysis (the most severely malnourished child), as we did on another occasion (HN, 1979). However, it is often difficult to decide which of two (or more) children is in the more severe condition. Of the 35 cases where mothers brought more than one child to the centre, in only 15 cases was a single child lowest on all three indices H-A, W-H and W-A. In the other 20 cases different siblings occupied the lowest position on different indicators.

[10] $t=1.96$; $df=53$; $p=.05$.

[11] t=0.95; df=53; p=.34.
[12] t=2.35; df=98; p=.02.
[13]Analysis of nutritional knowledge and preferences which was carried out for the MCH and FLT studies, revealed no interaction effects when results were broken down by area and income group (HN, 1980a: Appendices E–F; HN, 1982: Appendix K).
[14] As a further check, the relations between the formal education of the mother and the effects of the interventions were also analysed. No trends were discovered.

Chapter 8

[1] Hence one of the recommendations was that the FLT centres also admit women with severe domestic problems as a category in its own right, if only as a preventive measure.
[2] In fairness, it must also be pointed out that the evaluation is not concerned with any of the other activities of the Nutrition Field Workers, such as home visits and talks to various formal and informal groups elsewhere.
[3] This discussion of recent developments in impact evaluation is partly based on an earlier review article (Hoorweg, 1988).

References

Allen S.R. & Koral A.J. (1982). Food aid for supplementary feeding. In N.S. Scrimshaw & M.B. Wallerstein (Eds) **Nutrition policy implementation: Issues and experience.** New York: Plenum Press. Pp. 115–29.

Alleyne G.A.O., Hay R.W., Picou D.I., Stanfield J.P. & Whitehead R.G. (1977). **Protein-Energy Malnutrition.** London: Edward Arnold.

AMREF (1978). **Field work report on Kirathimo Family Life Training Centre, Kiambu, of the Ministry of Housing and Social Services, Kenya.** Nairobi: African Medical and Research Foundation.

AMREF (1979). **Field work report on Kirinyaga Family Life Training Centre, Kirinyaga, of the Ministry of Housing and Social Services, Kenya.** Nairobi: African Medical and Research Foundation.

AMREF (1980). **Field work report on Kigumo Family Life Training Centre, Murang'a, of the Ministry of Housing and Social Services, Kenya.** Nairobi: African Medical and Research Foundation.

Andersen K.B. (1977). **African traditional architecture: A study of the housing and settlement patterns of rural Kenya.** Nairobi: Oxford University Press.

Anderson M.A., Austin J.E., Wray J.D. & Zeitlin M.F. (1981). Supplementary feeding. In J.E. Austin & M.F. Zeitlin (Eds) **Nutrition intervention in developing countries.** Cambridge, Mass.: Oelgeschlager, Gunn & Hain. Pp. 25–48.

Anderson T.F. (1937). Kikuyu diet. **East African Medical Journal,** 14, 120–31.

Atlas of Kenya (1970). 3rd Ed. Nairobi: Survey of Kenya.

Austin J.E., Belding T.K., Brooks R., Cash R., Fisher J., Morrow R., Pielemeier N., Pyle D., Wray J.D. & Zeitlin M.F. (1981). Integrated nutrition programs and primary health care. In J.E. Austin & M.F. Zeitlin (Eds) **Nutrition intervention in developing countries.** Cambridge, Mass.: Oelgeschlager, Gunn & Hain. Pp. 123–36.

Austin, J.E. & Zeitlin M.F. (1981) (Eds). **Nutrition intervention in** developing countries. Cambridge, Mass.: Oelgeschlager, Gunn & Hain.

Bailey K.V. & Raba A. (1976). Supplementary feeding programmes. In G.H. Beaton & J.M. Bengoa (Eds) **Nutrition in preventive medicine.** Geneva: World Health Organization. WHO Monograph 62. Pp. 297–312.

Beaton G.H. (1982). Evaluation of nutrition interventions: Methodologic considerations. **American Journal of Clinical Nutrition,** 35, 1280–9.

Beaton G.H. & Bengoa J.M. (1976) (Eds). **Nutrition in preventive medicine.** Geneva: World Health Organization. WHO Monograph 62.

Beaton G.H. & Ghassemi H. (1982). Supplementary feeding programmes for young children in developing countries. **American Journal of Clinical Nutrition,** 35, 864–916 (Supplement 4).

Beaudry-Darisme M. & Latham M.C. (1973). Nutrition rehabilitation centres: An evaluation of their performance. **Journal of Tropical Pediatrics and Environmental Child Health,** 19, 299–332.

Beghin I.D. & Viteri F.E. (1973). Nutrition rehabilitation centres: An evaluation of their performance. **Journal of Tropical Pediatrics and Environmental Child Health,** 19, 404–16.

Bengoa J.M. (1976). Nutrition rehabilitation. In G.H. Beaton & J.M. Bengoa (Eds) **Nutrition in preventive medicine.** Geneva: World Health Organization. WHO Monograph 62. Pp. 321–34.

Benson, T.G. (1964). **Kikuyu–English dictionary.** Oxford: Clarendon Press.

Benson T.G. & Barlow A.R. (1975). **English–Kikuyu dictionary.** Oxford: Clarendon Press.

Bertin J., Hemardinquer J-J., Keul M. & Randles W.G.K. (1971). **Atlas of food crops.** The Hague: Mouton.

Blankhart D.M. (1974a). Human nutrition. In L.C. Vogel, A.S. Muller, R.S. Odingo, Z. Onyango & A. de Geus (Eds) **Health and disease in Kenya.** Nairobi: East African Literature Bureau.

Blankhart D.M. (1974b). **Regional names of foods in Kenya.** Nairobi: Medical Research Centre.

Block G. (1982). A review of validations of dietary assessment methods. **American Journal of Epidemiology,** 115, 492–505.

Bohdal M., Gibbs N.E. & Simmons W.K. (no date). **Nutrition survey and campaign against malnutrition in Kenya, 1964–1968.** Nairobi: Ministry of Health.

Bosley B. (1976). Nutrition education. In G.H. Beaton & J.M. Bengoa (Eds) **Nutrition in preventive medicine.** Geneva: World Health Organization. Pp. 277–96.

Brink E.W., Perera W.D., Broske S.P., Huff N.R., Staehling N.W., Lane J.M. & Nichaman M.Z. (1978). Sri Lanka Nutrition Status Survey, 1975. **International Journal of Epidemiology,** 7, 41–7.

Buijtenhuijs R. (1971). **Le mouvement Mau-Mau: Une revolte paysanne et anti-coloniale en Afrique Noire.** The Hague: Mouton.

Intervention in Child Nutrition (Kenya)

Burgess A. (1982). **Evaluation of nutrition interventions: An annotated bibliography and review of methodologies and results.** 2nd ed. Rome: Food and Agriculture Organization. Food and Nutrition Paper No. 24.

Buschkens W.F.L. & Slikkerveer L.J. (1982). **Health care in East Africa: Illness behaviour of the eastern Oromo in Hararghe (Ethiopia).** Assen: Van Gorcum.

Campbell D.T. & Stanley J.C. (1966). **Experimental and quasi-experimental designs for research.** Chicago: Rand McNally.

Campbell J.M. (1975). Report on an evaluation of the nutrition field worker programme of the Ministry of Health of the Government of Kenya. Nairobi: UNICEF Regional Office.

CBS (1972). Population projections by district, 1970–1980. **Kenya Statistical Digest,** 10, no. 3.

CBS (1976–1981). **Crop forecast surveys.** Nairobi: Central Bureau of Statistics.

CBS (1977). The rural Kenyan nutrition survey; February–March, 1977. **Social perspectives,** 2, no. 4.

CBS (1979a). **Report of the Child Nutrition Survey, 1978–1979.** Nairobi: Central Bureau of Statistics.

CBS (1979b). **Child nutrition in rural Kenya.** Nairobi: Central Bureau of Statistics.

CBS (1980). **Kenya fertility survey: 1977–1978. First report: Vol. 1.** Nairobi: Central Bureau of Statistics.

CBS (1981a). **The integrated rural surveys, 1976–1979: Basic report.** Nairobi: Central Bureau of Statistics.

CBS (1981b). **Kenya population census, 1979: Vol. 1.** Nairobi: Central Bureau of Statistics.

CBS (1983a). **Statistical abstract.** Nairobi: Central Bureau of Statistics.

CBS (1983b). **Third rural child nutrition survey, 1982.** Nairobi: Central Bureau of Statistics.

CBS (1983c). **Population projections for Kenya, 1980–2000.** Nairobi: Central Bureau of Statistics.

CBS/UNICEF (1984). **Situation analysis of children and women in Kenya, Section 4: The wellbeing of children.** Nairobi: Central Bureau of Statistics/UNICEF.

Church M.A. (1979). Dietary factors in malnutrition: Quality and quantity of diet in relation to child development. **Proceedings Nutrition Society,** 38, 41–9.

Collier P. & Lal D. (1980). **Poverty and growth in Kenya.** Washington: World Bank. Working Paper No. 389.

Cook R. (1971). Is hospital the place for treatment of malnourished children? **Environmental Child Health,** 17, 15–25.

Cook R. (1976). Immunization programmes in the context of prevention of malnutrition. In G.H. Beaton & J.M. Bengoa (Eds) **Nutrition in preventive medicine.** Geneva: World Health Organization. Pp. 268–76.

Cook T.D. & Campbell D.T. (1979). **Quasi-experimentation: Design and analysis issues for field settings.** Boston: Houghton Mifflin.

References

Cooper, R.A. & Weekes A.J. (1983). **Data, models & statistical analysis.** Oxford: Philip Allen.

Cranworth Lord (1939). **Kenya chronicles.** London: Macmillan.

CRS (1972). Interpreting growth records. Nairobi: Catholic Relief Services. Field Bulletin No. 15.

CRS-USCC (no date). Agreed policies and guidelines for the implementation of a preschool health program.

Cutting W.A.M. (1983). Nutrition rehabilitation. In D.S. McLaren (Ed) **Nutrition in the community.** New York: Wiley. Pp. 321–37.

FAO (1974). **Handbook on human nutritional requirements.** Rome: Food and Agricultural Organization.

Figa-Talamanca I. (1985). **Nutritional implications of food aid: An annotated bibliography.** Rome: Food and Agriculture Organization. Food and Nutrition Paper No. 33.

Fleuret P. & Fleuret A. (1980). Nutrition, consumption and agricultural change. **Human Organization,** 39, pp. 250–60.

FNSP (1985). Nutritional conditions at settlement schemes in Coast Province; Kwale and Kilifi District (Research Outline). Leiden: African Studies Centre. Food and Nutrition Studies Programme, Report No. 12.

Gachuhi J.M., Chege F.E. & Ascroft J. (1972). **Kirathimo model village of the Kenya Red Cross Society; An evaluation report.** Nairobi: Institute for Development Studies.

Garn S.M., Larkin F.A. & Cole P.E. (1978). The real problem with 1-day dietary records. **American Journal of Clinical Nutrition,** 31, 1114–16.

Gotzman H. (1986). Improved project design, monitoring and evaluation (some recent WFP experience). In **UNICEF/WFP Workshop: Food aid and the well-being of children in the developing world.** New York: UNICEF. Pp. 143–54.

Greer J. & Thorbecke E. (1983). Pattern of food consumption and poverty in Kenya and effects of food prices. Cornell University, mimeo.

Gussow J.D. & Contento I. (1984). Nutrition education in a changing world: A conceptualisation and selective review. **World Review of Nutrition and Dietetics,** 44, 1–56.

Haaga J., Mason J., Omoro F., Quinn V., Rafferty A., Test K. & Wasonga L. (1985). Child malnutrition in rural Kenya, A geographic and agricultural classification. **Ecology of Food and Nutrition,** 18, 297–307.

Habicht J-P. & Butz W.P. (1979). Measurement of health and nutrition effects of large-scale intervention projects. In R.E. Klein, M.S. Read, H.W. Riecken, J.A. Brown, A. Pradilla & C.H. Daza (Eds) **Evaluating the impact of nutrition and health programs.** New York: Plenum Press. Pp. 133–70.

Habicht J-P. & Mason J. (1983). Nutrition surveillance: Principles and practice. In D.S. McLaren (Ed) **Nutrition in the community.** New York: Wiley. Pp. 217–44.

Hartog A. den & Leemhuis E. (1985). Report on WFP-assisted project Bangla Desh 2226. The Hague: Ministry of Development Co-operation, mission report.

Hennigan K.M., Flay B.R. & Haag A. (1979). Clarification of concepts and terms commonly used in evaluative research. In R.E. Klein, M.S. Read, H.W. Rieken, J.A. Brown, A. Pradilla & C.H. Daza (Eds) **Evaluating the impact of nutrition and health programs.** New York: Plenum Press. Pp. 387–432.

Hitchings J.A. (1979). Indications of seasonal malnutrition in Kenya. Unpublished paper. Stanford University. Food Research Institute.

HN   See Hoorweg J. & Niemeijer R.

HNS   See Hoorweg J., Niemeijer R. & Steenbergen W. van.

Hoorweg J. (1983). The control of non-treatment variables: Necessity or illusion? In B. Schurch (Ed) **Evaluation of nutrition education in third world communities.** Bern: Hans Huber. Pp. 153–65.

Hoorweg J. (1988). Impact evaluation of child nutrition programmes. **Food Policy,** 13, 199–207.

Hoorweg J. & McDowell I. (1979). **Evaluation of nutrition education in Africa: Community research in Uganda, 1971–1972.** The Hague: Mouton.

Hoorweg J. & Niemeijer R. (1977). **Report on the Family Life Training Centres Bungoma, Busia, Kisumu, Kiambu and Murang'a.** Leiden: African Studies Centre. NIRP Report No. 4.

Hoorweg J. & Niemeijer R. (1978a). **Classification of foods among the Kikuyu.** Leiden: African Studies Centre. NIRP Report No. 7.

Hoorweg J. & Niemeijer R. (1978b). **Preferences of Kikuyu mothers for children's foods.** Leiden: African Studies Centre. NIRP Report No. 8.

Hoorweg J. & Niemeijer R. (1979). **Family Life Training Centres, Kenya, 1978.** Leiden: African Studies Centre. NIRP Report No. 10.

Hoorweg J. & Niemeijer R. (1980a). **The impact of nutrition education at three health centres in Central Province, Kenya.** Leiden: African Studies Centre. ASC Research Report No. 10.

Hoorweg J. & Niemeijer R. (1980b). **The nutritional impact of the Pre-School Health Programme at three clinics in Central Province, Kenya.** Leiden: African Studies Centre. ASC Research Report No. 11.

Hoorweg J. & Niemeijer R. (1980c). Preliminary studies on some aspects of Kikuyu food habits. **Ecology of Food and Nutrition,** 9, 139–50.

Hoorweg J. & Niemeijer R. (1982). **The effects of nutrition rehabilitation at three Family Life Training Centres in Central Province, Kenya.** Leiden: African Studies Centre. ASC Research Report No. 14.

Hoorweg, J., Niemeijer R. & Steenbergen W. van (1981). **Findings of the Nutrition Intervention Research Project.** Leiden: African Studies Centre. NIRP Report No. 15.

Hoorweg J, Niemeijer R. & Steenbergen W. van (1983). **Nutrition survey in Murang'a district, Kenya. Part 1: Relations between ecology, economic and social conditions and nutritional state of pre-school**

children. Leiden: African Studies Centre. ASC Research Report No. 19.
Hoorweg J., Niemeijer R. & Steenbergen W. van (1984). **Nutrition survey in Murang'a district, Kenya. Part 2: Nutritional cognition and the food consumption of pre-school children.** Leiden: African Studies Centre. ASC Research Report No. 21.
ICIHI (1985). **Famine: A man-made disaster?** London: Pan Books; Independent Commission on International Humanitarian Issues.
IDRC (1981). **Nutritional status of the rural population of the Sahel: Report of a working group, Paris, April 1980.** Ottawa: International Development Research Centre.
ILO (1983). **Increasing the efficiency of planning in Kenya: Concepts, methods and guidelines for reviewing performance and assessing impact.** Geneva: International Labour Office.

Jaetzold R. & Schmidt H. (1983). **Farm Management Handbook of Kenya, Vol IIB, Central Kenya.** Nairobi: Ministry of Agriculture/GTZ.
Jansen A.J., Horelli H.T. & Quinn V.J. (1987). **Food and nutrition in Kenya: A historical review.** Nairobi: UNICEF Regional Office.
Jelliffe D.B. (1966). **The assessment of the nutritional status of the community.** Geneva: World Health Organization. Monograph No. 53.

Kardjati S., Kusin J.A. & With C. de (1977). **Geographical distribution and prevalence of nutritional deficiency diseases in East Java, Indonesia.** Amsterdam: Royal Tropical Institute. East Java Nutrition Studies: Report 1.
Katona-Apte J. (1986). Women and Food Aid: A Developmental Perspective. **Food Policy, 11,** 216–22.
Keller W. (1983). Choice of indicators of nutritional status. In B Schurch (Ed) **Evaluation of nutrition education in third-world countries.** Bern: Hans Huber. Pp. 101–13.
Kerlinger F.N. (1973). **Foundations of behavioral research. 2nd ed.** London: Holt, Rinehart & Winston.
King M. (1966). **Medical care in developing countries.** Nairobi: Oxford University Press.
Klein R.A., Read M.S., Riecken H.W., Brown J.A., Pradilla A. & Daza C.H. (Eds) (1979). **Evaluating the impact of nutrition and health programs.** New York: Plenum Press.
Klein R.E., Townsend R.J., Praun A. & Fischer M. (1983). The practice of impact evaluation of nutrition education programs. In B. Schurch (Ed) **Evaluation of nutrition education in third-world countries.** Bern: Hans Huber. Pp. 136–51.
Korte R. (1969). The nutritional and health status of the people living in the Mwea-Tebere irrigation settlement. In H. Kraut & H.D. Cremer (Eds) **Investigations into health and nutrition in East Africa.** Munchen: Weltforum. Pp. 267–334.
Korte R. & Simmons W.K. (1972). The nutritional status of pre-school children in Kenya. **East African Medical Journal, 49,** 513–20.

Leakey L.S.B. (1977a, b, c). **The Southern Kikuyu before 1903. Vols 1, 2 & 3.** London: Academic Press.
Livingstone I. (1981). **Rural development, employment and incomes in Kenya.** Addis Ababa: ILO.
Maas M. (1986). **Women's groups in Kiambu: It is always good to have land.** Leiden: African Studies Centre. ASC Research Report No. 26.
Masai W. (1983). The nutritional status of Kenyans and major factors influencing it. In L.M. Wasonga & J.O. Otieno (Eds) **Proceedings of a workshop on Nutrition in Agricultural Development Projects.** Nairobi: Ministry of Economic Planning and Development. Pp. 3–59.
Mason J.B. & Habicht J.-P. (1984). Stages in the evaluation of ongoing programmes. In D.E. Sahn, R. Lockwood & N. Scrimshaw (Eds) **Methods for the evaluation of the impact of food and nutrition programmes.** Tokyo: United Nations University. Pp. 26–45.
Mason J.B., Habicht J.-P., Tabatabai H. & Valverde V. (1984). **Nutritional surveillance.** Geneva: World Health Organization.
Mbithi P.M. & Wisner B. (1972). **Drought and famine in Kenya: Magnitude and attempted solutions.** Nairobi: Institute for Development Studies. Discussion paper No. 144.
Meilink H. (1979). **Smallholder farming in Kiambu, Murang'a and Kirinyaga districts of Central Province, Kenya, with special reference to the three research areas.** Leiden: African Studies Centre. NIRP Report No. 11.
Middleton J. & Kershaw G. (1965). **The central tribes of the North-Eastern Bantu (revised ed.).** London: International African Institute.
Miller R.I. & Sahn D.E. (1984). Built-in evaluation systems for supplementary feeding programmes – why and how. In D.E. Sahn, R. Lockwood & N. Scrimshaw (Eds) **Methods for the evaluation of the impact of food and nutrition programmes.** Tokyo: United Nations University. Pp. 265–87.
MoEPCA (1979). **Development Plan, 1979–1983. Part 1.** Nairobi: Ministry of Economic Planning and Community Affairs.
MoFEP (1970). **Kenya population census, 1969, Vol. 1.** Nairobi: Ministry of Finance and Economic Planning.
MoHSS (1976–79). **Annual Reports, Family Life Training Programme, 1976–1979.** Nairobi: Ministry of Housing and Social Services.
MoHSS (1980) **A guide for Family Life Training facilitators.** Nairobi: Ministry of Housing and Social Services.
Munger S.J. (1983). The generalizability of evaluation protocols for nutrition education. In B. Schurch (Ed) **Evaluation of nutrition education in third-world communities.** Bern: Hans Huber. Pp. 183–226.
Muriuki G. (1974). **A history of the Kikuyu, 1500–1900.** Nairobi: Oxford University Press.

Nelson, H.D. (Ed) (1984). **Kenya: A country study.** Washington: American University. Foreign Area Studies.
Niemeijer R., Geuns M., Kliest T., Ogonda V. & Hoorweg J. (1985).

Nutritional aspects of rice cultivation in Nyanza Province, Kenya.
Leiden: African Studies Centre. FNSP Report No. 14.
Niemeijer R., Geuns M., Kliest T., Ogonda V. & Hoorweg J. (1988)
Nutrition in agricultural development: The case of irrigated rice
cultivation in West Kenya. **Ecology of food and nutrition.** (In press).
NIRP (1976). Nutrition intervention and environment: research proposal.
Leiden: African Studies Centre. NIRP Report.
NIRP (1977). **A short dictionary of Kikuyu names of foods, meals and
drinks.** Leiden: African Studies Centre. NIRP Report No. 3.
NIRP (1978). Revised research plan. Leiden: African Studies Centre.
NIRP Report No. 5.

Ojany F.F. & Ogendo R.B. (1973). **Kenya: A study of physical and
human geography.** Nairobi: Longman.
O'Keefe P. (1978). Gakara, a study in the development of
underdevelopment. London: PhD Thesis.
Oomen H.A.P.C., Blankhart D.M. & Mannetje W. (1984). Growth
pattern of pre-school children. In J.K. van Ginneken & A.S. Muller
(Eds) **Maternal and child health in rural Kenya.** London: Croom Helm.
Pp. 183–96.
Oomen H.A.P.C., Jansen A.A.J. & Mannetje W. (1979). Growth
pattern of rural Akamba pre-school children. **Tropical and
Geographical Medicine,** 31, 422–39.
Orr J.B. & Gilks J.L. (1931). **Studies of Nutrition: The physique and
health of two African tribes.** Medical Research Council, special report
155. London: HMSO.

Paterson A.R. (1943). Health and Agriculture. **East African Medical
Journal,** 20, 194–200.
PBFL/FAO (1973). **Proceedings of a seminar on survey of programmes
concerned with family life in Kenya.** Nairobi: Kenya National Council
of Social Services.
PCI (1980). Kenya Food for Peace; Title II Evaluation. Washington:
USAID/Practical Concepts Incorporated.
Pinstrup-Andersen P. (1983). Export crop production and malnutrition.
Food and Nutrition, 9, 7–14.
Platt B.S. (1962). **Tables of representative values of foods commonly used
in tropical countries** (revised ed.). Medical Research Council, special
report No. 302. London: HMSO.
Poskitt E.M.E. (1979). Report on Kenyan Family Life Training
Programme. London: British Council.
Procter R.A.W. (1926). The Kikuyu market and Kikuyu diet. **Kenya
Medical Journal,** 3, 15–22.

Riecken H.W. (1979). Practice and problems of evaluation: A conference
synthesis. In R.E. Klein, M.S. Read, H.W. Riecken, J.A. Brown,
A. Pradilla & C.H. Daza (Eds) **Evaluating the impact of nutrition and
health programs.** New York: Plenum Press. Pp. 363–86.

Rodrigues V. (1972). Food production and diet: A case study at
Githunguri. MA Thesis: University of Nairobi.
Rogers P. (1979). The British and the Kikuyu 1880–1905: A reassessment.
Journal of African History, 20, 255–69.
Routledge W.S. & Routledge K. (1910). **With a prehistoric people: The
Akikuyu of British East Africa.** London: Cass (reprint 1968).
Sahn D.E. (1985). Methods for evaluating the nutritional impact of food
aid projects: Lessons from past experience. **Food and Nutrition Bulletin,**
6, 1–14.
Sahn D.E., Lockwood R. & Scrimshaw N. (Eds) (1984). **Methods for
the evaluation of the impact of food and nutrition programmes.** Tokyo:
United Nations University.
Sahn D.E. & Pestronk R.M. (1981). **A review of issues in nutrition
program evaluation.** Washington: USAID. Program Evaluation
Discussion Paper No. 9.
Saxe L. & Fine M. (1981). **Social experiments: Methods for design and
evaluation.** Beverly Hills: Sage Publications.
Schofield S. (1979). **Development and the problems of village nutrition.**
London: Croom Helm.
Schurch B. (Ed) (1983). **Evaluation of nutrition education in third-world
communities.** Bern: Hans Huber.
Schurch B. & Wilquin L. (1982). **Nutrition education in communities of
the third world: An annotated bibliography.** Lausanne: Nestle
Foundation.
Scrimshaw N.S. (1982). Programs of supplemental feeding and weaning
food development. In N.S. Scrimshaw & M.B. Wallerstein (Eds)
Nutrition policy implementation: Issues and experience. New York:
Plenum Press. Pp. 101–11.
Shack K.W. (Ed) (1977). **Teaching nutrition in developing countries or,
the joys of eating dark green leaves.** Santa Monica: Meals for Millions
Foundation.
Sinclair H.M. & Howat G.R. (1980). **World nutrition and nutrition
education.** Oxford: Oxford University Press.
Siswanto A.W., Kusnanto J.H. & Rohde J.E. (1980). Comparison of
nutritional results of clinic based and village based weighing programs.
Paediatrica Indonesia, 20, 93–103.
Sorrenson M.P.K. (1967). **Land reform in the Kikuyu country.** Nairobi:
Oxford University Press.
Stamp P. (1975). Perceptions of change and economic strategy among
rural Kikuyu women of Mitero, Kenya. **Rural Africana,** 29,
19–43.
Steenbergen W. van, Kusin J.A. & Jansen A.A.J. (1984). Food
consumption of pre-school children. In J.K. van Ginneken & A.S.
Muller (Eds). **Maternal and child health in rural Kenya.** London:
Croom Helm. Pp. 167–82.
Sterkenburg J.J. (1978). **Housing conditions in rural Kiambu, Kenya.**
University of Utrecht: Dept. of Geography of Developing Countries.
Stevens C. (1979). **Food aid and the developing world: Four African case
studies.** London: Croom Helm.

References

Suchman E.A. (1967). **Evaluative research: Principles and practice in public service and social action programmes.** New York: Russell Sage Foundation.

Thomson A. (1986). Food aid as income transfer. In M.J. Forman (Ed) **Nutritional aspects of project food aid.** Rome: United Nations, ACC/SCN (FAO). Pp. A38–A46.

Tignor R.L. (1976). **The colonial transformation of Kenya: The Kamba, Kikuyu and Maasai from 1900 to 1939.** Princeton: Princeton University Press.

Timmons R.J., Miller R.I. & Drake W.D. (1983). **Targeting: A means to better intervention.** Ann Arbor: Community Systems Foundation.

Timmons R., Miller R. & Drake W.D. (1986). Selecting participants for community nutrition interventions in developing countries. In M.J. Forman (Ed) **Nutritional aspects of project food aid.** Rome: United Nations, ACC/SCN (FAO). Pp. A1–A20.

Tosh J. (1980). The cash-crop revolution in tropical Africa: An agricultural reappraisal. **African Affairs,** 79, 79–94.

Underwood B.A. (Ed) (1983). **Nutrition intervention strategies.** New York: Academic Press.

UNICEF (1985). **The state of the world's children.** London: Oxford University Press.

USAID (1976). **Liberia: National Nutrition Survey.** Washington: Agency for International Development, Office of Nutrition.

USAID (1978a). **Sierra Leone: National Nutrition Survey.** Washington: Agency for International Development: Office of Nutrition.

USAID (1978b). **United Republic of Cameroon: National Nutrition Survey.** Washington: Agency for International Development: Office of Nutrition.

Waterlow J. (1976). Classification and definition of protein-energy malnutrition. In G.H. Beaton & J.M. Bengoa (Eds). **Nutrition in preventive medicine.** Geneva: World Health Organization. WHO Monograph 62. Pp. 530–55.

Weiss C.H. (1972). **Evaluation research: Methods of assessing program effectiveness.** Englewood Cliffs N.J.: Prentice Hall.

Wenlock R.W. (1980). Nutritional risk and the family environment in Zambia. **Ecology of Food and Nutrition,** 10, 79–86.

WHO (1985). **Energy and protein requirements.** Geneva: World Health Organization. Technical Report 724.

World Bank (1986). **The World Bank Atlas – 1986.** Washington.

Zeitlin M. (1981). Intervention evaluation. In M.F. Zeitlin & C.S. Formacion. **Nutrition intervention in developing countries. Study 2: Nutrition education.** Cambridge, Mass.: Oelgeschlager, Gunn & Hain.

Zeitlin M.F. & Formacion C.S. (1981). Nutrition education. In J.E. Austin & M.F. Zeitlin (Eds) **Nutrition intervention in developing countries.** Cambridge, Mass.: Oelgeschlager, Gunn & Hain. Pp. 49–72.

Index

Page numbers followed by 'n' refer to notes.
Page numbers in *italics* refer to boxes, figures or tables, textual matter may
also occur.